Blueprints for Health

An
ILLUSTRATED
ADVENTURE
in
HUMAN
ANATOMY

Written and Illustrated by Kate Sweeney

Anatomical Chart Company, Skokie, Illinois

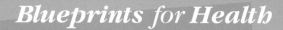 Lippincott Williams & Wilkins
a Wolters Kluwer business
Philadelphia • Baltimore • New York • London
Buenos Aires • Hong Kong • Sydney • Tokyo

Written and Illustrated by: Kate Sweeney

Art Director and Designer: Lisa Ott

Medical Editor: William E. Burkel, M.A., Ph.D

Editors: Nancy Liskar and Randy Stott

Published in the United States in 2002 by
The Anatomical Chart Company
A division of Lippincott Williams & Wilkins
A Wolters Kluwer Company
8221 Kimball Avenue,
Skokie, Illinois 60076-2956

Second Edition

ISBN: 1-58779-49O-X
Library of Congress Card Number: 2002102054

Printed and bound in the United States of America.

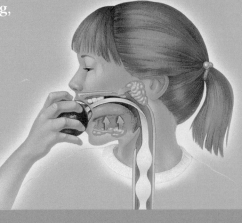

Table of
CONTENTS

Your Skeletal System 1

Your Muscular System 7

Your Nervous System 13

Your Circulatory System . . . 19

Your Respiratory System . . . 25

Your Digestive System 31

Your Eyes 37

Your Ears 43

Your Taste and Smell 49

Glossary 55

References 56

Your SKELETAL *System*

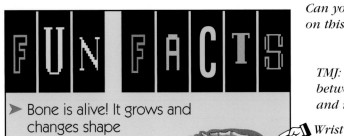

FUN FACTS

➤ Bone is alive! It grows and changes shape throughout your life. Your skeleton is one-third living tissues and two-thirds water and minerals. The minerals calcium and phosphorus give your bones strength and make them hard.

➤ Your bones are 4 times as strong as concrete. They can be stronger than steel, but they weigh 4 times less! A 2-inch block of bone can hold the weight of an elephant!

➤ Babies are born with over 300 bones, but adults have only 206 bones. What happens to the other 94 bones? As you grow, some smaller bones join to make larger bones.

➤ Measure yourself when you first get out of bed in the morning and then right before you go to bed at night. What do you find? People are taller in the morning than in the evening. This is because the discs between the bones in the spine squash down during the day and go back to their full height when you sleep.

Your RIB CAGE

The rib cage is made of twelve ribs on each side. Ribs 1–7 are "true ribs." Each attaches directly to the sternum by individual pieces of cartilage. Ribs 8–10 are "false ribs." Their individual pieces of cartilages come together and attach to the 7th rib. Ribs 11 and 12 are called "floating ribs," and they don't attach to the sternum or other ribs.

Joints

Can you find your joints? Look for the "☞" on this page and touch your joints.

TMJ: joint between skull and mandible ☞

☞ *Wrist*

Shoulder ☞

Sternum (breast bone)

Floating ribs

Spine (backbone)

Pelvis

Hip ☞

The **femur** *(thigh bone) is the largest bone in your body.*

Knee ☞

Ankle ☞

The **cranium** (skull) *looks like one bone, but it's made of 22. The only bone that moves is the* **mandible** (jaw bone).

Clavicle (collar bone)

Scapula (shoulder blade)

Rib cage

Humerus

☞ *Elbow*

Radius

Ulna

Carpals (wrist bones)

Metacarpals (Palm bones)

Phalanges (finger bones)

Each hand has 27 bones. Over one quarter of the bones in your body are in your hands!

Patella (kneecap)

Tibia (shin bone)

Fibula

Calcaneus (heel bone)

Tarsals

Metatarsals

Phalanges (toe bones)

Stegosaurus

Whale

Frog

Bat

Bones give SUPPORT

Without your skeleton, your body would collapse in a heap. Each bone has a special job to do. The bones in your arms and legs are long and narrow to help you reach things and run fast. The bones in your pelvis are strong and round like a bowl to protect your insides.

Cervical (1–7) (neck vertebrae)

1 2 3 4 5 6 7

Thoracic (1–12) (rib cage vertebrae)

1 2 3 4 5 6 7 8 9 10 11 12

Lumbar (1–5) (lower back vertebrae)

1 2 3 4 5

Your Spine

or backbone, is made of 33 bones called vertebrae.

Vertebrae are stacked on top of each other like blocks. They let you bend and twist your back.

The **spinal cord,** the main nerve in your body, runs down a tunnel in the stack of vertebrae. The bony surrounding vertebrae protect the spinal cord.

Each vertebra is joined to its neighbor by an **Intervertebral disk.** The vertebral disk is a rubbery pad that cushions your spine when you move. Each disk has two parts: a strong rubbery outside and a jelly-like center.

Bonus

At the end of your spine are 2 more sections of vertebrae: the **sacrum** (made of 5 fused bones) and the **coccyx** or tail bone (made of 4 fused bones).

Joints allow MOVEMENT

A joint is the place where two bones meet. The joints between bones let us move. Some joints move in many directions, like your shoulder joint. Some joints don't move at all, like the joints in your skull! Some joints work together and let you bend over or to the side, like your spine. Where else do you have joints that move?

Bones give PROTECTION

The bones of your skull are strong and round like a helmet to protect your brain. Your ribs make a cage to protect your heart and lungs.

The smallest bones in your body are inside your skull! They are called the **malleus, incus,** and **stapes** bones, and they help you hear. These bones could fit on a dime!

Malleus (hammer)

Incus (anvil)

Stapes (stirrup)

(2X enlarged)

Gorilla

Human

Elephant

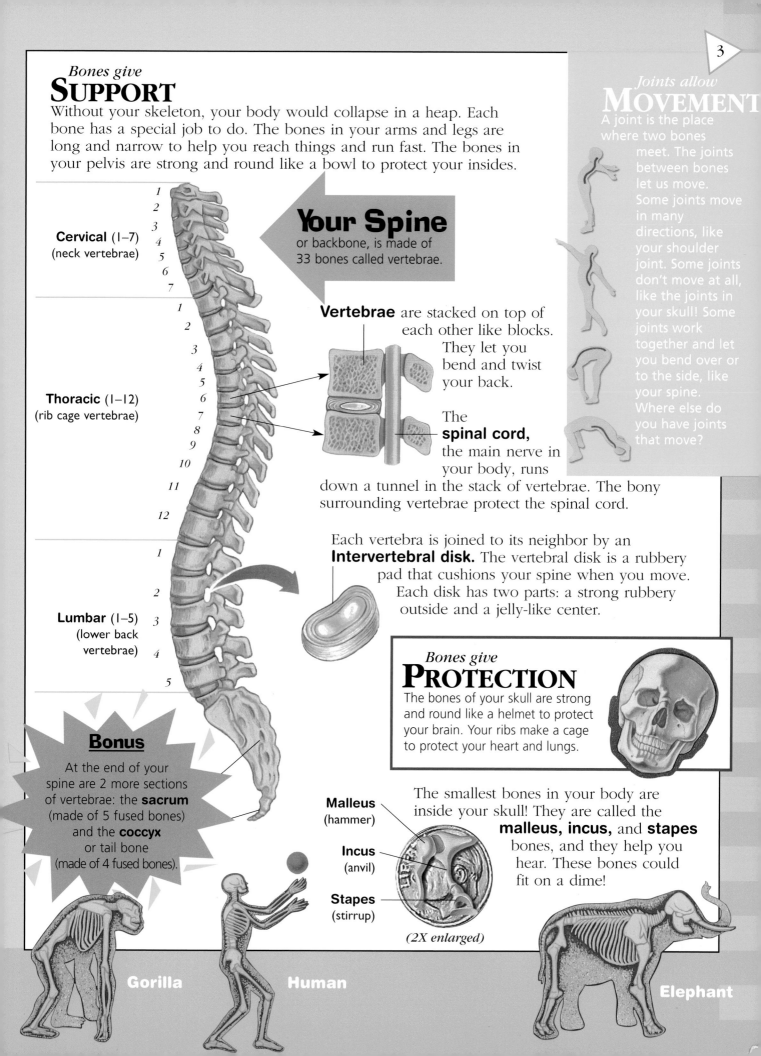

Growing
BONES

Bones start out as soft, bendable cartilage. The cartilage is slowly replaced by bone cells and minerals as you grow. Each bone is made of several parts at first. The parts join together, or fuse, as you grow older. The bones need a good diet to grow and stay healthy. Eating food that contains calcium and phosphorus helps your bones to be their best.

Cartilage

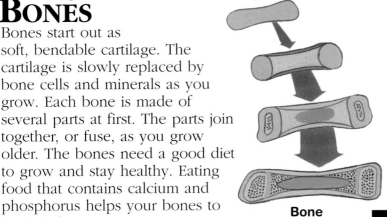

Bone

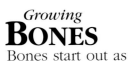

*Your nose is made of **cartilage** not bone! Cartilage is a strong, bendable. rubbery tissue. Your ears are made of cartilage too. Can you wiggle your nose and ears?*

X-rays are energy waves used to take pictures of your bones and cartilage. Children have cartilage bones and adults have hard bones.

Child **Adult**

X - R A Y

Inside Your Bones

Your bones are not solid. Bone is made of many kinds of tissue.

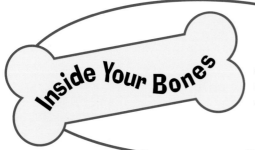

Cartilage covers the ends of the bones at the joints. It is a rubbery tissue that cushions and protects bones as they rub together.

Spongy bone is very light and strong. It is filled with tiny holes, like a sponge. Spongy bone is found at the ends of long bones like your femur, or inside chunky bones like your spine.

Red marrow is found in the spongy parts of your bones. Red marrow makes red blood cells, an important part of blood.

Yellow marrow is stored in the center of long bones like your femur. Yellow marrow holds fat used for energy by your body.

Compact bone is strong, dense outer bone. Bone cells live inside compact bone and make new bone. The new bone grows in rings, like the rings in a tree trunk. Blood vessels in each ring carry energy and blood in and out of the bone.

Here is what one bone cell looks like inside the tiny mineral cave it lives in.

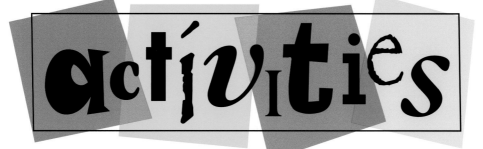

activities

Match Up!!

Your bones have a scientific name and a common name. Can you match up the scientific names on the left with the common names on the right?

Scientific name	Common name
Cranium	Thigh bone
Mandible	Shin bone
Scapula	Arm bone
Clavicle	Jaw bone
Sternum	Shoulder blade
Humerus	Collar bone
Femur	Skull
Patella	Finger bones
Tibia	Kneecap
Calcaneus	Breast bone
Pelvis	Heel bone
Phalanges	Hips

Here are some bone words missing a few letters. Can you find the words in this chapter to solve the puzzle?! (example – co**cc**yx).

```
T       R   S           L   L
H   U       K       L       S
    P       E   L   V   I   S
    F       L   E   M       R
P   A   C   T   E   L   A   X
    C       O   C   C   Y   X
    I       N           S
```

Look for this symbol 👉 *on page 2–*
You can touch your skeleton!

• Put your fingers on the side of your face right in front of your ears. Move your jaw up and down. You can feel your TMJ, the joint where your jaw fits into your skull.

• Find the point of your scapula at the outer corner of your shoulder. Does it move when you lift your arm up and down? Can you touch your clavicle? Follow it from end to end.

• Feel the edge of your rib cage at your waist. Follow it up to the center of your chest where it joins your sternum. Breathe in and out. Does your rib cage move?

• Feel the knobs at either side of the end of your humerus. The tingling feeling you notice when you hit your "funny bone" is made by a nerve at your elbow, not by your bone.

• Feel the end of your ulna at the back of your elbow. You can feel the ends of your arm bones, the radius and ulna, at the sides of your wrist.

• Find your patella, or kneecap, and gently wiggle it. It is connected by tendons to the muscles above your knee and to your tibia below.

• Your "ankle bones" are really the ends of the tibia and fibula, the bones in your lower leg. You can feel them at the outside of your ankle.

Bigger and Bigger!!!

Girls may keep growing until they are 20 years old. Boys can keep growing until they are 25 years old.

When boys are 9 years old, they are 75% of their adult height. They will grow 33.3% taller before they stop.

Girls reach 75% of their adult height at 7 years old.

Can you figure out how tall you may get?

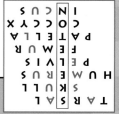

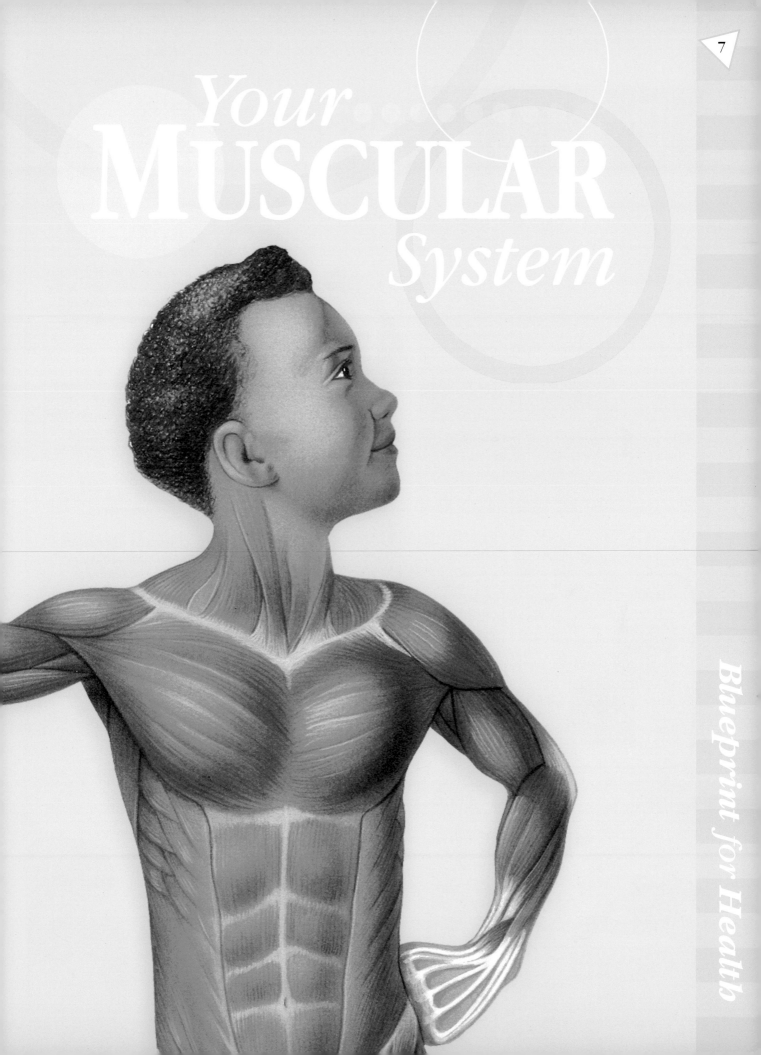

Your MUSCULAR System

FUN FACTS

- Muscles are made of one-quarter protein and three-quarters water. They make up almost one-half of your total body weight.

- You have more than 600 muscles in your body. The longest muscle is the sartorius muscle, in your leg. It stretches from on top of your hip to below your knee. The biggest muscle is the one you sit on–the gluteus maximus! Some of your strongest muscles are in your tongue. The fastest muscles are the ones that make your eyes blink.

- You never stop moving, even when you sleep. Muscles keep your heart beating, your lungs breathing, and your digestion working. Even your eyes move in your sleep!

Pupil

In the light

In the dark

You even have a muscle in your eye! This tiny muscle controls the size of your pupil. Can you see this muscle at work?

Your MUSCLES

Muscles shorten, or **contract**, to move bones. When they contract, they bulge and get hard.

Touch your thumb to your little finger on one hand. Can you see and feel the muscles on either side of your palm? They help you grab and hold things.

Turn your head to one side. The long, straight muscle that runs from behind your ear to the beginning of your collar bone is the **Sternocleidomastoid***. It helps turn your head.*

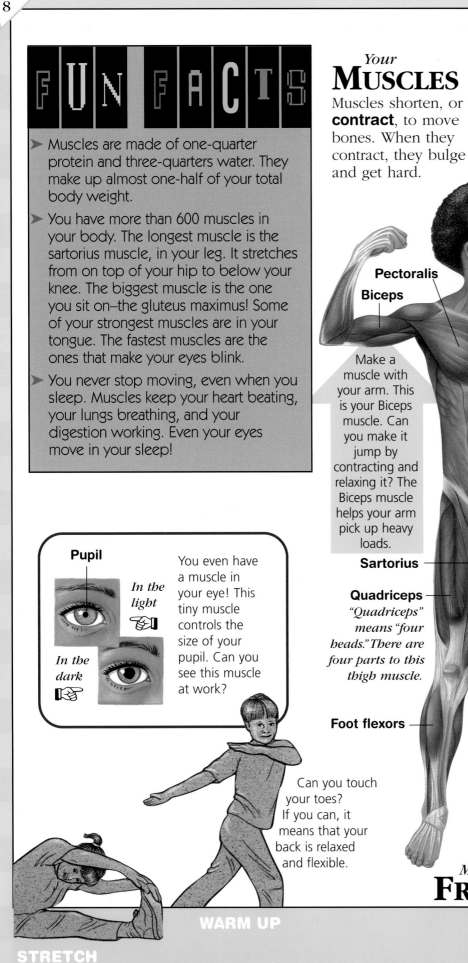

Pectoralis

Biceps

Make a muscle with your arm. This is your Biceps muscle. Can you make it jump by contracting and relaxing it? The Biceps muscle helps your arm pick up heavy loads.

Deltoid
"Deltoid" means "shaped like a triangle." Can you see the triangle this muscle makes?

Hand & Finger extensors

Rectus abdominis
Can you see your rectus abdominis muscle when you do sit-ups? This muscle helps keep your body straight and protects your back.

Sartorius

Quadriceps
"Quadriceps" means "four heads." There are four parts to this thigh muscle.

Patella
(kneecap bone)
Stand up and contract the muscles on the front of your thigh. Can you feel your kneecap move?

Foot flexors

Can you touch your toes? If you can, it means that your back is relaxed and flexible.

Muscles in **FRONT**

STRETCH

WARM UP

Tips for Healthy Muscles

EAT RIGHT

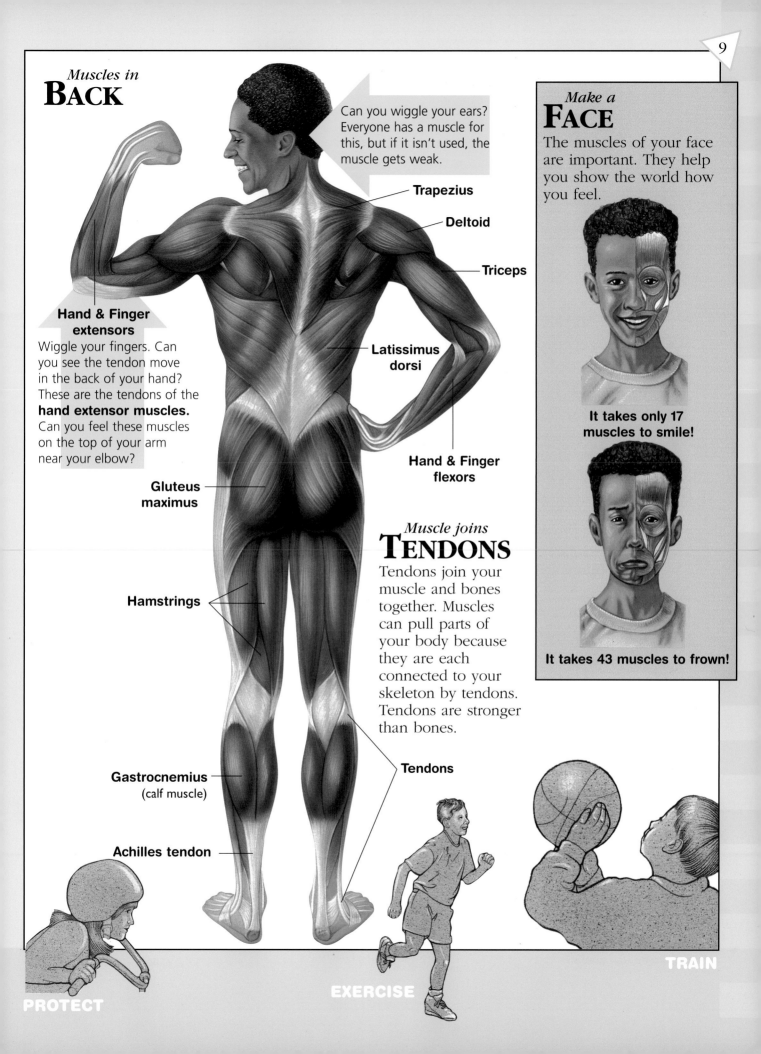

Muscles in
BACK

Can you wiggle your ears? Everyone has a muscle for this, but if it isn't used, the muscle gets weak.

Trapezius

Deltoid

Triceps

Latissimus dorsi

Hand & Finger extensors
Wiggle your fingers. Can you see the tendon move in the back of your hand? These are the tendons of the **hand extensor muscles.** Can you feel these muscles on the top of your arm near your elbow?

Hand & Finger flexors

Gluteus maximus

Muscle joins
TENDONS
Tendons join your muscle and bones together. Muscles can pull parts of your body because they are each connected to your skeleton by tendons. Tendons are stronger than bones.

Hamstrings

Tendons

Gastrocnemius (calf muscle)

Achilles tendon

Make a
FACE
The muscles of your face are important. They help you show the world how you feel.

It takes only 17 muscles to smile!

It takes 43 muscles to frown!

PROTECT

EXERCISE

TRAIN

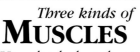

Three kinds of
MUSCLES

Your body has three kinds of muscles. Each has a special job to do.

Skeletal muscle is the main type in your body. It connects to your bones and helps you move. You can tell this kind of muscle what to do, which makes it a "voluntary" muscle.

Smooth muscle is the main type inside your organs. It's at work right now in your stomach, intestines, lungs and blood vessels. It works all the time, without you noticing or telling it what to do. This makes it an "involuntary" muscle.

Cardiac muscle is found only in your heart. This special kind works all the time, without you thinking about it. It automatically contracts faster when you exercise and slows down when you rest or sleep. This makes it an "involuntary" muscle.

Inside your
MUSCLES

1. Each muscle is made from thousands of cells called **muscle fibers**. The muscle fibers are bundled together into strands called **fascicles**.

2. A single muscle fiber can be up to a foot long, but very narrow. Each muscle fiber is made from bundles of proteins called **myofibrils**.

3. A myofibril is made of two kinds of proteins called **filaments**. The **thick filament** is named **myosin**. The **thin filament** is named **actin**. The filaments are grouped together in long rows inside each myofibril.

4. When the signal to contract reaches the thick and thin filaments, they slide past each other in rows.

5. When this happens, the muscle becomes shorter, or **contracts**. The muscle relaxes when the signal stops and the filament rows return to original length.

Muscle

Fasciculus

Muscle fibers

Myofibril

Thin filament

Thick filament

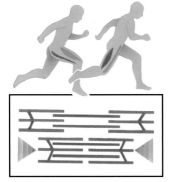

Muscles can only **contract** or pull. After one muscle contracts and moves a part of your body, another muscle needs to contract to move your body back. When you run, your legs move back and forth. Muscles on the front and back of your legs are taking turns contracting.

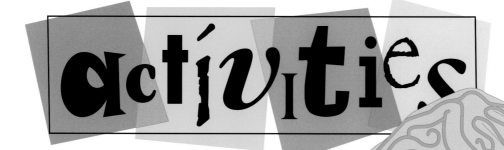

See who's **stronger**, boys or girls

Try this challenge and see who wins—boys or girls!
You'll need a straight-back chair, a boy and a girl.

1 Stand an arm length away from a wall, facing it
with your feet together.
2 Have your friend place the chair between you
and the wall.
3 Lean forward and put your forehead on
the wall.
4 Hang your arms straight down by the sides
of the chair.
5 Grab the chair and lift it as you try to
stand straight up.

What happens if you're a **girl?**
What happens if you're a **boy?**

*Girls can lift the chair up,
but boys won't be able to!*

WHY?

This is because a boy's center
of balance is higher than a girl's.
There's not enough weight in
the lower half of a boy's body
to counteract the weight of
the chair when bending over
to pick it up. A girl's center
of gravity is lower than a
boy's. This allows her
to balance the weight
of the chair with the
weight of her
lower body.

MUSCLE MAZE

Start Here!

Finish Here!

What are goose bumps?

Each hair on your body has a tiny muscle attached to it. The hair stands up straight when the muscle contracts. The "bumps" are these contracted muscles just under the skin. Goose bumps appear when you are cold because hairs that stick up can trap more warm air between them. Like a cat's fur on a cold day, your hairs are "fluffing up" to trap heat and keep you warm.

Why do you shiver when you get cold?

Besides moving your body, muscles have another important job to do—keeping you warm. Muscle movement makes heat in your body as muscle fuel is burned up. If you are standing still too long in the cold, your body will take over and make tiny movements—shivers—to make more heat with your muscles, which will keep you warm.

Why do muscles get tired?

Muscles are fueled from the energy you get from the food you eat and oxygen you breathe. When muscles work hard, they burn up this "fuel" quickly. The blood replaces the used up fuel from food energy stored in fat and increased oxygen from breathing harder. Sometimes muscles work so hard that the blood can't keep up with their need for more oxygen. Muscles keep moving, burning up food energy with no air. This creates lactic acid, which makes muscles feel sore and tired. When you stop and rest, the blood can bring more oxygen and take away lactic acid. Your muscles feel better.

Your NERVOUS *System*

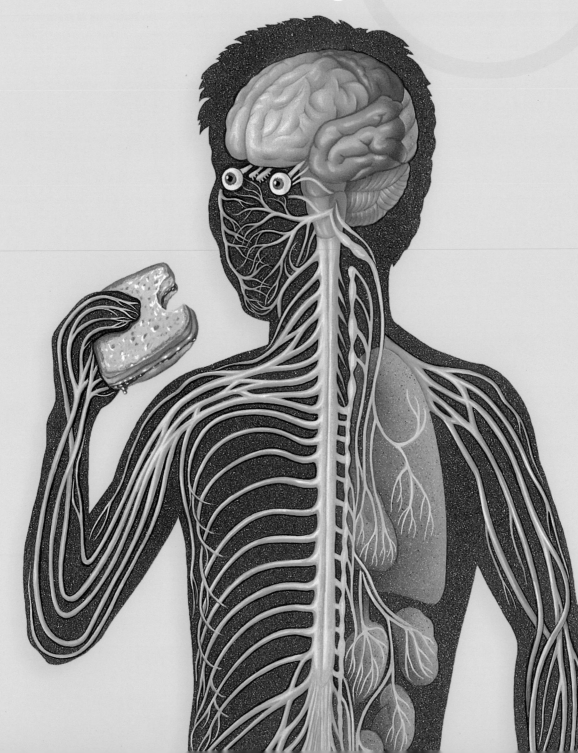

Your
BRAIN AND NERVES

Your nervous system is the main communication system of your body. Your brain and nerves help to control all your activities. If you had to think about breathing, digesting, and the beating of your heart, you wouldn't get another thing done! So your nervous system has two parts. One part runs automatically—the **autonomic system.** It controls breathing, digesting, and heart rate without you being aware of it. The other part is the **somatic system.** Under your control, it directs your muscles, thinking, and speech.

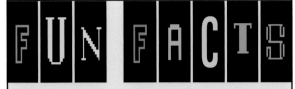

- ➤ Your nerves can send signals at more than 200 miles per hour!
- ➤ Your brain is 80% water!
- ➤ Your brain stops growing when you are 15. But learning never stops! Your brain's nerve cells make new connections throughout life.
- ➤ Your brain uses as much power as a 10—watt light bulb!
- ➤ There are probably 10 billion to 100 billion nerve cells in your brain.
- ➤ Each nerve cell in your brain can have up to 250,000 connections to other nerve cells!
- ➤ Humans have the biggest brain compared to body size of any animal that ever lived.

Automatic Reflexes
A reflex is a quick reaction to something sudden. Your muscles act before your brain knows what's happening. You step on something sharp and your foot pulls back before you can think! What's happening here?

1. The signal "Ouch!!" from your sensory nerve cell travels in an instant to your spinal cord.
2. It connects directly to the nerves controlling the muscles of your foot.
3. The motor nerve sends an instant message back to your muscles—"Pull back!"
4. At the same time, the sensory nerve message is traveling to your brain. It takes a little longer to arrive. When it does, you think "Wow!! That could have hurt!"

Lobes in each half of your brain control different activities.

Frontal Lobe—personality, reasoning, speech, muscles
Parietal Lobe—speech, sensory signals
Occipital Lobe—vision
Temporal Lobe—hearing, speech, understanding

This side shows the **Autonomic System.** *It controls organs like your liver, lungs, heart, stomach and intestines.*

This side shows the **somatic system.** *It directs your muscles.*

WHAT'S SO FUNNY?
Your "funny bone" is really a nerve! The ulnar nerve in your arm curves around your elbow. If you bump your elbow, the nerve gets pinched against the bone and sends a big signal —YOW!— to your brain.

Learned Reflexes
When you first learn to catch a ball or ride a bike, you don't always do it well. Practice creates more connections between nerve cells. This helps you make a bigger and better pathway for nerve impulses. Soon the pathway is so strong, you don't have to think about it, you just do it.

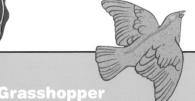

How do these brains compare to yours?

Fish

Frog

Grasshopper

Bird

Your BRAIN

The brain makes you aware. It works much faster than any computer! Billions of nerve cells get messages from the outside world, decide what to do, and tell the body to act. The cerebrum is where you think and decide on actions. Memories are stored here. The outer layer, or cortex, of the cerebrum is folded to make room for more nerve cells. The cerebrum is divided into halves called **hemispheres.**

The **center of the brain** controls basic actions like instincts, emotions, hunger and thirst. It is a pathway between the brain and the spinal cord. The **brainstem** controls automatic actions like breathing, heart rate, digestion, coughing, sneezing and swallowing. **Cerebellum** means "small brain." It processes signals traveling between the brain and spinal cord. It automatically makes your muscles work together smoothly.

LEFT BRAIN OR RIGHT BRAIN

Each half of your brain is not identical. The left half controls speech, math information, emotions, and artistic creativity. In each person one side is more in control than the other. About 90% of right-handed people are "left-brained." The rest and left-handed people are "right-brained."

Drugs Are Phoney Baloney!

Deep in the center of your brain is a "pleasure center." Chemical nerve messengers in your brain send messages to this center. These messages affect how much you eat and drink, how you feel, what you choose for play, and who you have a crush on! Addictive drugs destroy the brain's own chemical nerve messengers and replace them with fake messengers. When the drug high wears off, drug users 'crash.' They need the drug to feel good because their own chemical messengers are ruined. Drug addicts can't feel good naturally.

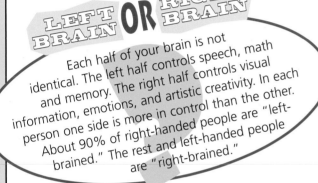

Your SPINAL CORD

The spinal cord is a pathway for nerves between your brain and your body.

31 pairs of **spinal nerves** leave the **spinal cord.** They spread out through every part of your body, collecting sensory signals and sending out motor signals.

The end of the spinal cord is called the **cauda equina,** or "horse's tail." Can you guess why?

Build a Better Brain!

Scientists think people are born with a range of "possible intelligence." How smart you become depends on how much you 'exercise' your brain. You can't add brain cells. You can add connections between cells. This happens when you learn and practice. Adding connections makes your brain faster and more powerful.

SPINAL NERVES

SPINAL CORD

CAUDA EQUINA

Dog

Gorilla

Elephant

THREE KINDS OF NERVE CELLS

There are three main kinds of nerve cells. Each has a different job.

Inside your NERVE CELLS

Your body is full of electricity. Your nerve cells carry electricity. They can instantly send messages to the other cells of your body. Your nerve cells are sending and getting thousands of messages from other cells right now!

NERVE GLUE

You have nerve glue in your brain! Nerve cells called **neuroglia** help hold other nerve cells together. There are 10 times as many "nerve glue" cells in your brain as there are "thinking" nerve cells.

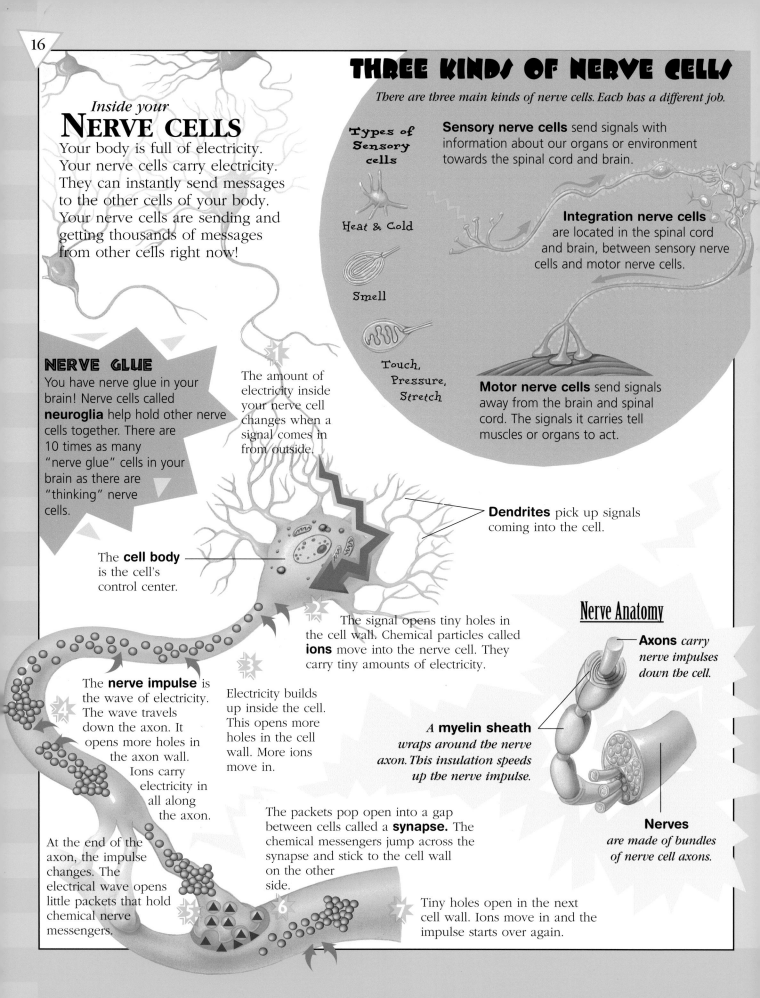

Types of Sensory cells

Heat & Cold

Smell

Touch, Pressure, Stretch

Sensory nerve cells send signals with information about our organs or environment towards the spinal cord and brain.

Integration nerve cells are located in the spinal cord and brain, between sensory nerve cells and motor nerve cells.

Motor nerve cells send signals away from the brain and spinal cord. The signals it carries tell muscles or organs to act.

The amount of electricity inside your nerve cell changes when a signal comes in from outside.

The **cell body** is the cell's control center.

Dendrites pick up signals coming into the cell.

The signal opens tiny holes in the cell wall. Chemical particles called **ions** move into the nerve cell. They carry tiny amounts of electricity.

The **nerve impulse** is the wave of electricity. The wave travels down the axon. It opens more holes in the axon wall. Ions carry electricity in all along the axon.

Electricity builds up inside the cell. This opens more holes in the cell wall. More ions move in.

At the end of the axon, the impulse changes. The electrical wave opens little packets that hold chemical nerve messengers.

The packets pop open into a gap between cells called a **synapse.** The chemical messengers jump across the synapse and stick to the cell wall on the other side.

Tiny holes open in the next cell wall. Ions move in and the impulse starts over again.

Nerve Anatomy

Axons *carry nerve impulses down the cell.*

A **myelin sheath** *wraps around the nerve axon. This insulation speeds up the nerve impulse.*

Nerves *are made of bundles of nerve cell axons.*

activities

FOOL YOUR BRAIN!

1. Cross your arms in front, elbows straight.
2. With palms together, fold your fingers together and lock them.
3. Bend your elbows, then pull your hands under and up to your chest.
4. Ask a friend to point to one finger without touching it.
5. Try to move just that finger. How easy is it? Have your friends try! How do they do?

DO THE JERK!

1. Have a friend sit on the edge of a chair or table with his or her legs dangling in the air.
2. Hit one of the legs just below the knee with the side of your hand. Be quick, not hard.
3. When you hit the right spot, what happens? You've sent a message to your friend's spinal cord and it answers by making his or her leg do a little kick!

That Funny Floating Feeling

1. Stand in an open doorway.
2. Press your arms straight against the doorway.
3. Push as hard as you can for as long as you can—until your arms shake—2 or 3 minutes.
4. What happens when you move out of the doorway? Your nerves are still sending messages to your brain to "Push up!" even after you stop!

Memory Training Contest

1. Form a circle with several friends.
2. The first person begins the story: "I packed my bag with a _____," filling in the blank with the name of something.
3. The next person goes on: "I packed my bag with a _____ and a _____," repeating the first thing and adding one of his or her own.
4. Go around the circle, each person adding a thing to the list after repeating from memory all the things on the list from before.
5. Drop out if you miss something. How do people work to remember items on the list? What details do they use to remember something?

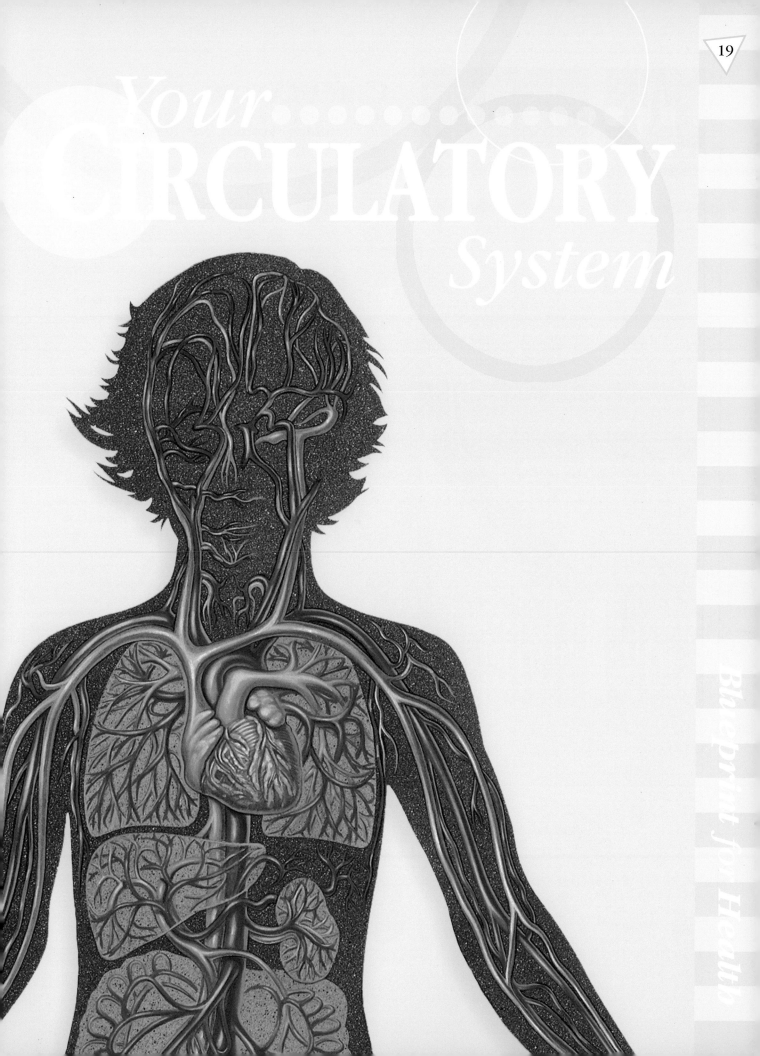

Your CIRCULATORY System

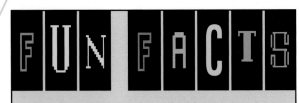

FUN FACTS

- Inside every cubic inch of your body are 80 million red blood cells.

- If all your red blood cells were laid end to end they would stretch more than two times around the earth!

- Blood is 80% water.

- Every pound of excess fat contains 200 miles of capillaries. Your heart has to work harder to push blood through those extra miles!

- Your body has over 70,000 miles of blood vessels. They could stretch around the earth over 2 ½ times!

- You have 9 feet of blood vessels in every square inch of skin on the back of your hand.

- There are over 1,500 miles of capillaries in your lungs.

- Your heart beats 100,000 times each day. That's over 36 million times a year.

- Your heart pumps over 40 tons of blood a day, more than the weight of 6 full-grown elephants! That adds up to over 75,000 pints of blood in a single day.

- As an adult you have about 5 liters of blood. That's more than two big soda pop bottles!

Each beat of your heart blood is pushed through your vessels. When you feel your pulse, you are really feeling blood moving in your vessels.

Find Your Pulse Points!
Can you find places on your body where you feel your pulse? Look for the "finger" sign and try it!

Your
CIRCULATORY SYSTEM

The heart, blood and blood vessels are called the **circulatory system.** They deliver what your body and cells need to live. Your heart pumps blood through your blood vessels. Your blood carries food energy, oxygen and special chemical messengers. It helps get rid of waste and protects you from germs and infections. Your blood helps keep you warm.

(body diagram labels: 6, 3, 8, 2, Lung, Heart, Lung, Liver, 5, 7, Kidney, 4, Intestines, 6, 6)

RUN A RACE *with your* **BLOOD!**
This race will last only 45 seconds, so get ready!

1 *Blood moves out of your heart and rushes to your lungs.*

2 *In your lungs, red blood cells load up on oxygen and run back to your heart.*

3 *Blood gets a big push out of your heart and into arteries.*

4 *Your blood races around your intestines. It pauses to pick up food energy. The blood then heads to the liver.*

5 *In the liver, food energy is repackaged for the body to use. Your blood picks up the newly packaged food energy and delivers it to your cells.*

6 *Blood speeds energy and oxygen to every cell in your body. Waste products made by your cells are picked up by your blood.*

7 *Your blood zooms through your kidneys. They filter and clean your blood.*

8 *Blood returns to your heart and then rushes back to your lungs, where carbon dioxide is dumped off.*

Sponge

Frog

Grasshopper

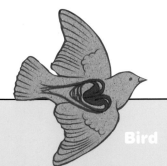

Bird

Your HEART

The heart sits in the middle of your chest. It's about as big as your fist. The muscles in the wall of your heart are the most powerful in your body. They work twice as hard as other muscles.

Your heart is like two pumps working side-by-side. Each side has two rooms, or chambers. The top chamber is the atrium, and the bottom is the ventricle. They are separated by valves that control what direction the blood goes. The muscular walls squeeze the sides of the chambers, pushing blood through your heart.

Follow these arrows to see where blood goes inside the **Heart!**

The sound of your **heartbeat** is the sound of your heart valves slamming shut with every beat. Your heart beats once a second.

Aorta (to your body)
Pulmonary artery (to your lungs)
Pulmonary veins (from your lungs)
Left atrium
Bicuspid valve
Left ventricle
Heart wall muscles
Descending aorta (to your body)

Superior vena cava (from your body)
Pulmonary Valve
Aortic Valve
Right atrium
Tricuspid Valve
Right ventricle
Inferior vena cava

Your BLOOD CELLS

Blood cells are made in the center of your bones! Your bone marrow is a blood-making factory. All blood cells come from one type of cell called a **stem cell.** Stem cells grow and change into each of the special cells in your blood. Young blood cells live in your bone marrow. When they are fully grown, they enter your blood and start working.

BONE MARROW

Red blood cells
carry oxygen to your cells. You have over 30 trillion red blood cells in your body right now! Each red blood cell lives for 120 days. Making 75,000 trips through your blood stream in its lifetime. Inside your Red Blood Cells are tiny particles called **hemoglobin.** Iron in hemoglobin makes your blood look red. Each red blood cell holds 270 million hemoglobin molecules. They carry 4 oxygen molecules each.

Platelets
are made of small pieces of larger blood cells. They travel through your blood helping to form scabs over your cuts and control bleeding.

White blood cells
help to fight infections. You have five kinds of white blood cells. Each kind does a special job. Most patrol your body, hunting for invaders. When they find one, they attack and destroy the invader. These "protector" cells work hard and live a short, dangerous life. They are quickly replaced by new cells made in your bone marrow.

Plasma
is the clear liquid part of your blood. It's over half of the stuff that makes up your blood . Plasma is 90% water. And the rest is important particles like minerals and special proteins that help plug up cuts, fight diseases, and make your blood thick. Plasma carries food energy to your cells.

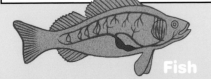
Fish
Earthworm
Dog

Inside your
BLOOD VESSELS

First, the power of your pumping heart pushes your blood through vessels called **arteries.** Arteries have thick muscular walls. They help your heart squeeze blood out to all your cells.

Your arteries get smaller and smaller. Your smallest vessels are called **capillaries.** They reach every cell in your body. They are ten times finer than a human hair! Capillaries can be so narrow that red blood cells squeeze through them single file!

Artery

Capillaries

Vein

Valve

Your
VEINS

The capillaries join back together to make larger vessels called **veins.** Veins have thin walls with few muscles. They have valves to help move blood back to your heart.

Your
CAPILLARIES

Capillaries have gaps in their walls. Food energy, water and oxygen in your blood can slip through the gaps and jump into your cells. And waste products can squeeze into the capillaries.

White blood cells

Red blood cells

Oxygen

Capillary wall

Food energy

Carbon dioxide

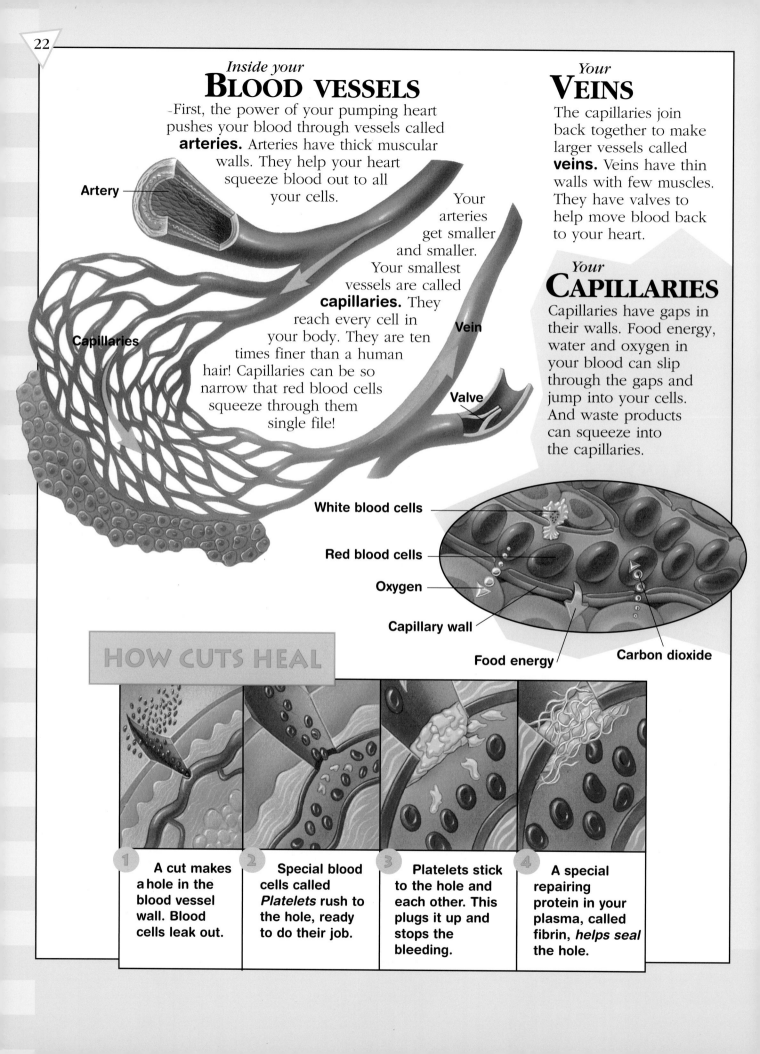

HOW CUTS HEAL

1 A cut makes a hole in the blood vessel wall. Blood cells leak out.

2 Special blood cells called *Platelets* rush to the hole, ready to do their job.

3 Platelets stick to the hole and each other. This plugs it up and stops the bleeding.

4 A special repairing protein in your plasma, called fibrin, *helps seal* the hole.

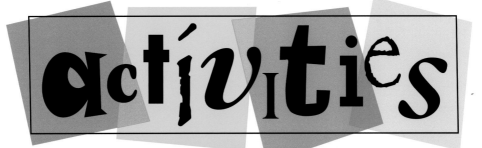

Test yourself on how the blood travels!

Use the information found in this chapter and the illustration under "answers" to help you match up the sentence with the correct letter.

_____ 1. What pumps your blood?

E 2. Where do the pulmonary arteries carry your blood?

_____ 3. Your blood gets what from your lungs?

_____ 4. Which side of the heart pumps the blood out to the body?

_____ 5. What is the largest artery in the body?

_____ 6. Blood travels through these three types of vessels.

_____ 7. Blood from the body returns to the heart through which veins?

ANSWERS (match these letters with questions 1 - 7)

A Inferior and superior vena cava

B Aorta

C The heart

D Arteries, capillaries and veins

E The lungs

F Left side

G Oxygen

Numbers on this illustration relate to each question

1.C 2.E 3.G 4.F 5.B 6.D 7.A

COUNT YOUR HEART RATE

Use a watch with a second hand. Press gently on a pulse point. You should feel a soft beat. Count the number of beats in 15 seconds. Multiply by 4.

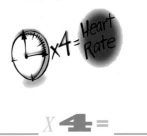

___ X **4** = ___

This number is the total beats per minute, or heart rate. Compare heart rates of friends, family and pets. What do you find? What is your heart rate in the morning, after you eat, exercise, study, get excited, or watch TV?

SEE YOUR BLOOD VESSELS

Use a mirror. Look underneath your tongue. Can you see big vessels just under the surface? Pull down your lower eyelid. There are tiny blood vessels on the inside. Look for tiny vessels in the whites of your eyes. Can you see little blue veins at the inside of your wrist?

HOW HARD DOES YOUR HEART WORK?

Squeeze a tennis ball once a second for two minutes. Can you do it? That's how hard your heart works!

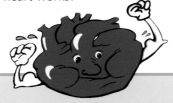

LISTEN TO YOUR HEART

Get a length of tubing and a plastic pop bottle. Cut the top half off the plastic bottle and attach the tube to the neck of the bottle. Place the bottle end gently on the center of your friend's chest. Hold the other end of the tube to your ear. What do you hear?

Your RESPIRATORY *System*

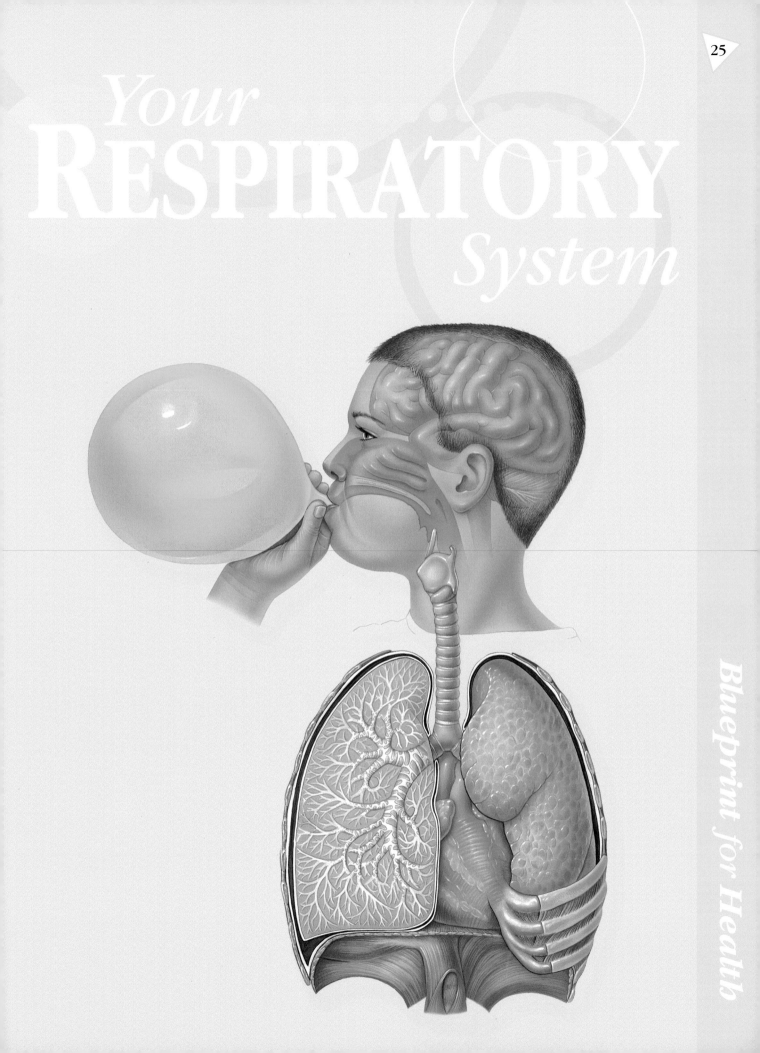

How do you BREATHE?

Air contains oxygen gas. The cells of your body need oxygen to make energy. To get the oxygen to each cell in your body, you first inhale into your lungs. The oxygen passes out of your lungs and into your blood. The oxygen gas combines inside your cells with nutrients in the food you eat. The oxygen and nutrients burn together. This makes the energy your cells and body need to run.

Feel the little hairs in your nostrils. They trap particles before you breathe them into your nose. When particles get in, you sneeze!

Your BRAIN

The brain controls breathing. It checks the amount of gases in your blood. When there is too much carbon dioxide gas, your brain automatically tells your diaphragm and ribcage to move. This brings air in and out of your lungs. You don't have to think about this.

Throat
Epiglottis
Larynx
Trachea

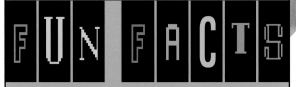

FUN FACTS

- Your lungs are each the size of a loaf of bread. They hold about 3 quarts of air. Only 19% of the air we breathe is oxygen.
- You take over 20,000 breaths a day!
- There are over 30,000 tubes in the lungs, which have over 300 million air sacs attached to them.
- Your lungs are the only organs in the body that can float! They are spongy and lighter than water because of all the air-filled sacs in them.
- If you took all the air sacs in your lungs and stretched them out flat, you could have enough material to cover 100 people from head to toe.
- A sneeze makes an air blast of up to 100 miles per hour; a cough can make a blast of 400 miles per hour!

Your NOSE

The nose filters and warms air you breathe. The inside of your nose is covered by **mucous membrane.** As air moves over it, this sticky lining traps particles. The twisty shape of the membrane helps to heat up the air.

Your THROAT

Your mouth and nose connect together at the back of your throat, or **pharynx.** Your throat connects to your windpipe, or **trachea.** At the top of the trachea is a trap door called the **epiglottis.** It keeps food out of your trachea.

top view of larynx

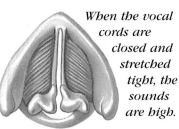

When the vocal cords are closed and stretched tight, the sounds are high.

When the vocal cords are apart and looser, the sounds are low.

Your VOICE

Your voice comes from your voice box, or **larynx,** at the top of your trachea. Your vocal cords stretch across the inside of your larynx. When air passes over the **vocal cords,** they vibrate. This makes a sound.

You can feel your larynx vibrate as you talk! Put your fingertips on the front of your neck. Talk! Can you feel a difference between high and low sounds?

How do these living creatures breathe?

Tadpole: *Gills*

Frog: *Lungs and Skin*

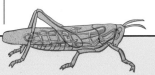

Grasshopper: *Air Tubes*

Your LOWER RESPIRATORY SYSTEM

Your TRACHEA

The trachea, or windpipe, connects your throat to your lungs. It is about 4 inches long. Stiff cartilage rings give it support. The trachea divides in two as it enters the lung. Each side is called a **bronchus.** Each bronchus divides into many tiny tubes called **bronchioles.** Your lungs have more than 30,000 bronchioles!

Your LUNGS

You have two lungs, one on each side of your chest. Inside, the **bronchus** connects to **bronchioles** and then **alveoli.** Outside, the **pleura** covers your lungs. The pleura is very thin and slippery. It helps your lungs move easily inside your rib cage. Your rib cage protects your lungs.

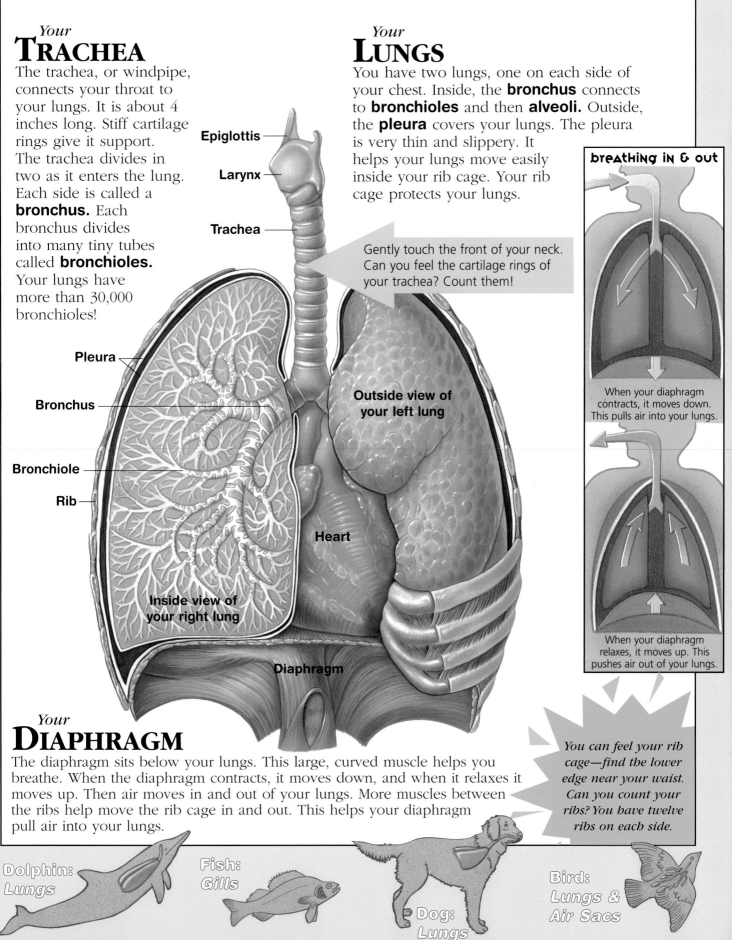

Epiglottis

Larynx

Trachea

Gently touch the front of your neck. Can you feel the cartilage rings of your trachea? Count them!

Pleura

Bronchus

Bronchiole

Rib

Outside view of your left lung

Inside view of your right lung

Heart

Diaphragm

breathing in & out

When your diaphragm contracts, it moves down. This pulls air into your lungs.

When your diaphragm relaxes, it moves up. This pushes air out of your lungs.

Your DIAPHRAGM

The diaphragm sits below your lungs. This large, curved muscle helps you breathe. When the diaphragm contracts, it moves down, and when it relaxes it moves up. Then air moves in and out of your lungs. More muscles between the ribs help move the rib cage in and out. This helps your diaphragm pull air into your lungs.

You can feel your rib cage—find the lower edge near your waist. Can you count your ribs? You have twelve ribs on each side.

Dolphin: *Lungs*

Fish: *Gills*

Dog: *Lungs*

Bird: *Lungs & Air Sacs*

Inside your
LUNGS

Your lungs are made of thousands of tiny air sacs called **alveoli.** They fill up with air when you inhale. Their thin walls let oxygen easily pass through to your blood in the vessels surrounding the alveoli.

Here is a special close up picture of healthy alveoli.

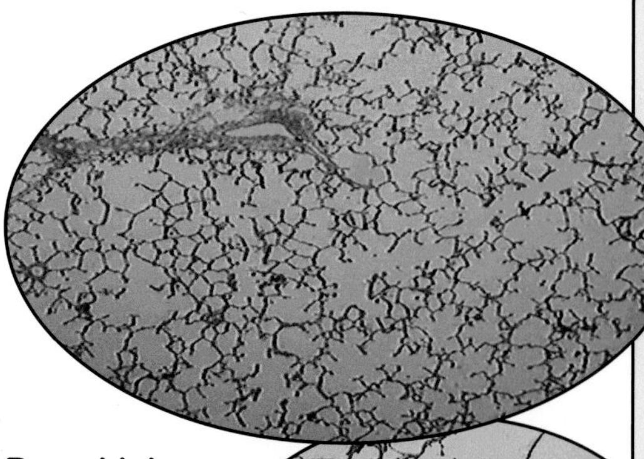

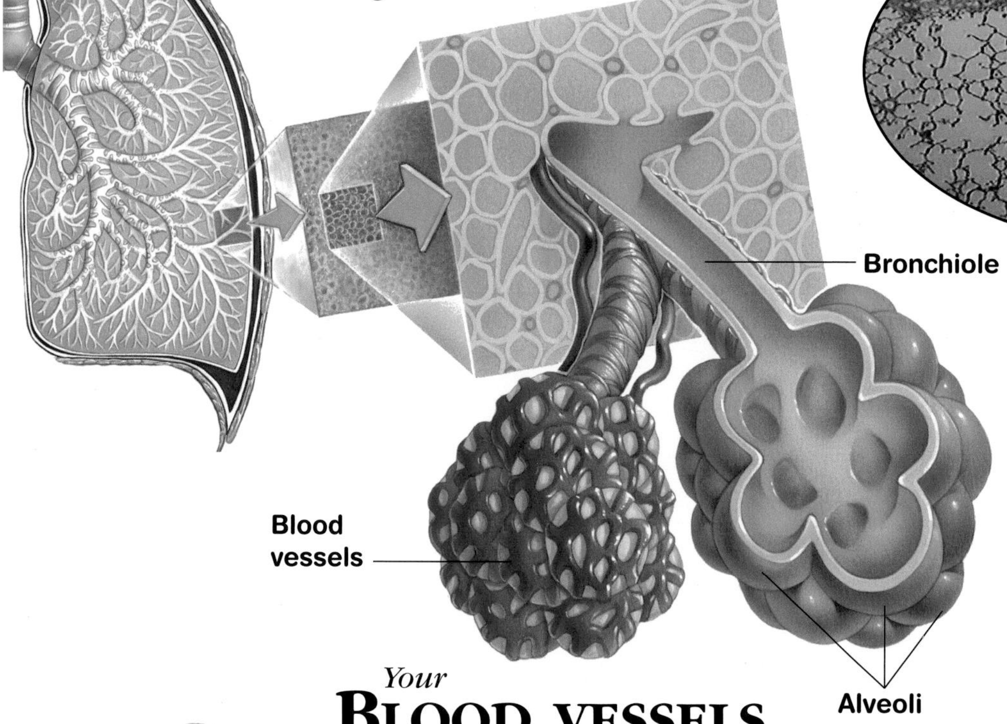

Bronchiole

Blood vessels

Alveoli

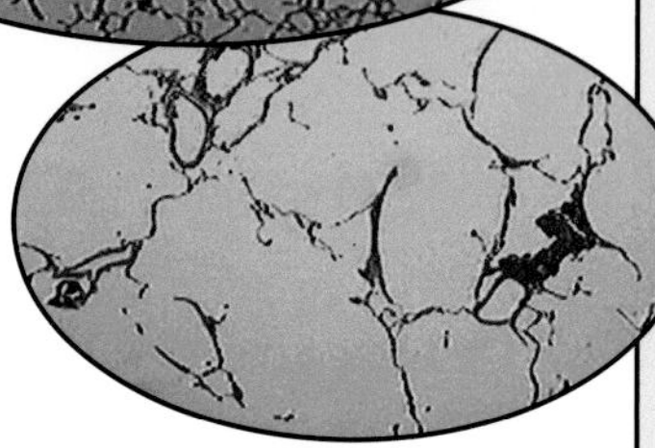

Here is a picture of alveoli that have been damaged by cigarette smoke.

Your
BLOOD VESSELS

carry red blood cells to and from the alveoli. Red blood cells carry oxygen and carbon dioxide inside them. Each one can carry over one billion oxygen molecules! They travel through your blood vessels to deliver oxygen to all of your cells. They also pick up carbon dioxide & waste products to bring back to the alveoli.

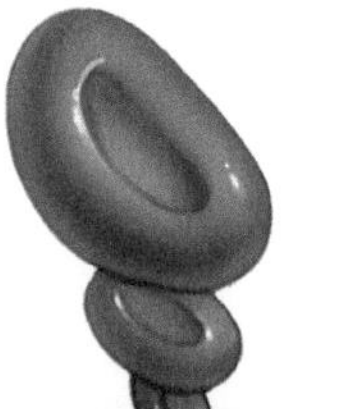

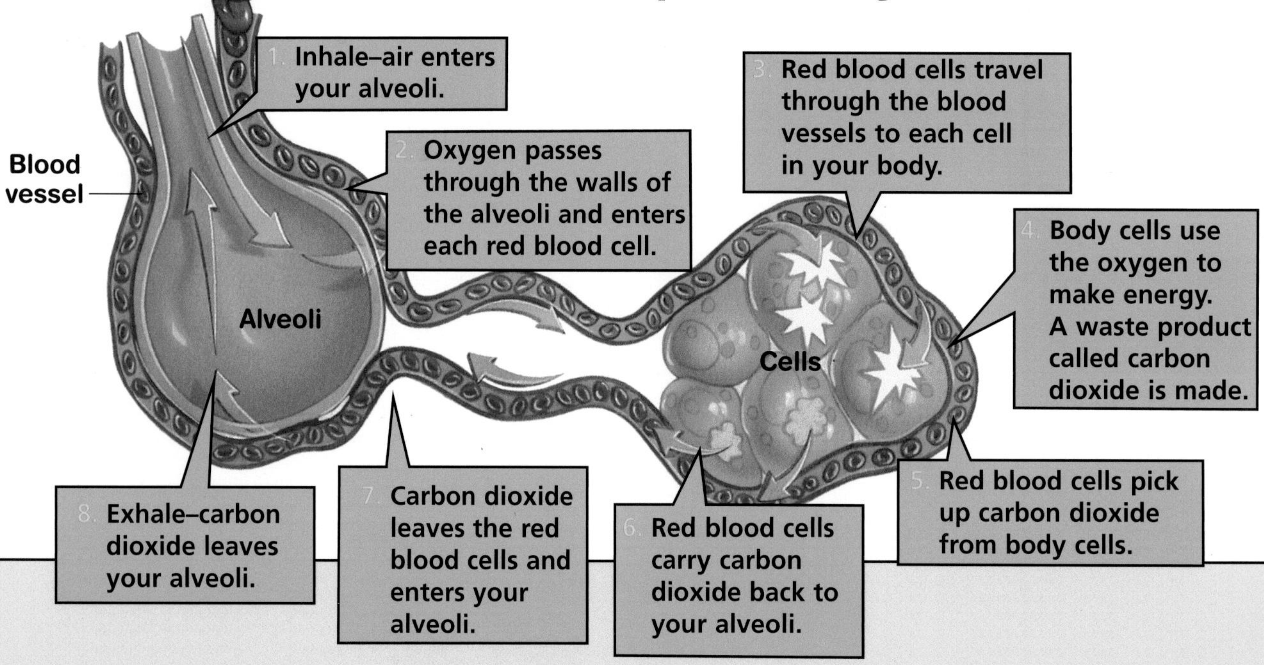

1. Inhale–air enters your alveoli.

2. Oxygen passes through the walls of the alveoli and enters each red blood cell.

3. Red blood cells travel through the blood vessels to each cell in your body.

4. Body cells use the oxygen to make energy. A waste product called carbon dioxide is made.

5. Red blood cells pick up carbon dioxide from body cells.

6. Red blood cells carry carbon dioxide back to your alveoli.

7. Carbon dioxide leaves the red blood cells and enters your alveoli.

8. Exhale–carbon dioxide leaves your alveoli.

Blood vessel

Alveoli

Cells

activities

MAKE A MODEL OF YOUR LUNGS!

YOU NEED:
- a plastic soda bottle
- 2 balloons
- a piece of modeling clay
- a plastic drinking straw
- a rubber band
- scissors

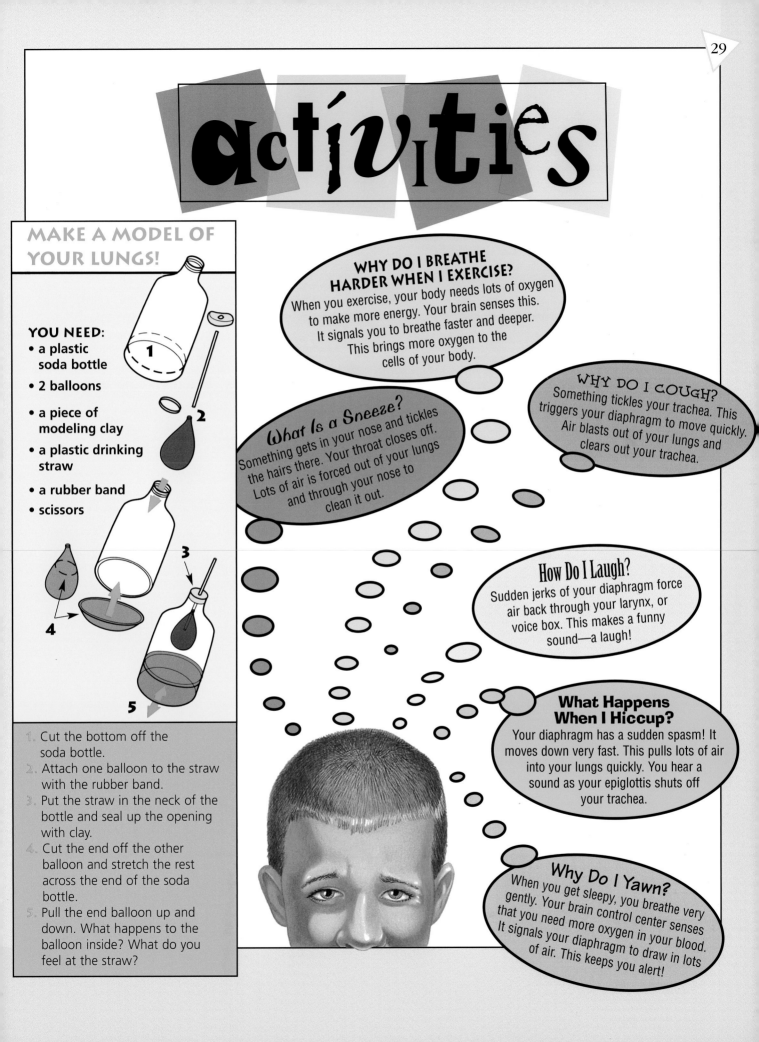

1. Cut the bottom off the soda bottle.
2. Attach one balloon to the straw with the rubber band.
3. Put the straw in the neck of the bottle and seal up the opening with clay.
4. Cut the end off the other balloon and stretch the rest across the end of the soda bottle.
5. Pull the end balloon up and down. What happens to the balloon inside? What do you feel at the straw?

WHY DO I BREATHE HARDER WHEN I EXERCISE?
When you exercise, your body needs lots of oxygen to make more energy. Your brain senses this. It signals you to breathe faster and deeper. This brings more oxygen to the cells of your body.

What Is a Sneeze?
Something gets in your nose and tickles the hairs there. Your throat closes off. Lots of air is forced out of your lungs and through your nose to clean it out.

WHY DO I COUGH?
Something tickles your trachea. This triggers your diaphragm to move quickly. Air blasts out of your lungs and clears out your trachea.

How Do I Laugh?
Sudden jerks of your diaphragm force air back through your larynx, or voice box. This makes a funny sound—a laugh!

What Happens When I Hiccup?
Your diaphragm has a sudden spasm! It moves down very fast. This pulls lots of air into your lungs quickly. You hear a sound as your epiglottis shuts off your trachea.

Why Do I Yawn?
When you get sleepy, you breathe very gently. Your brain control center senses that you need more oxygen in your blood. It signals your diaphragm to draw in lots of air. This keeps you alert!

Your DIGESTIVE *System*

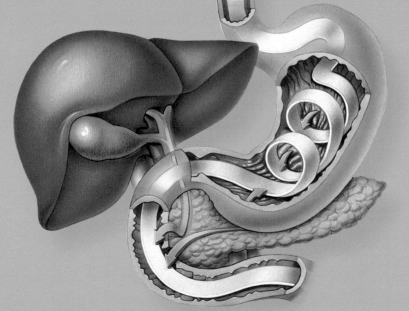

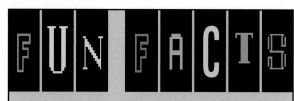

FUN FACTS

- ➤ Adults eat about 3 pounds of food a day.
- ➤ Borborygmus (Bore-bore-RIG-mus) is a word for the sounds your digestive system makes when it is working!
- ➤ Junk food is food that has lots of calories and extra fat, but not very many useful ingredients. When you eat junk food, you don't get a good supply of vitamins, energy and building blocks.
- ➤ Over half your body weight is water! Even though some foods seem solid, they contain lots of water. Lettuce is 96% water!

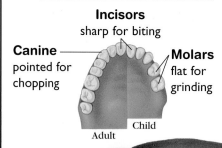

Enamel
Dentin
Gums
Nerve
Root
Bone

TEETH ARE DIFFERENT SHAPES FOR DIFFERENT JOBS:

Incisors
sharp for biting

Canine
pointed for chopping

Molars
flat for grinding

Adult   Child

Your TEETH

The teeth are made of hard tissues called **dentin** and **enamel.** The roots sit in your jaw bones and are covered by your gums. Healthy gums protect teeth.

Two sets of teeth grow during life: a baby set and a permanent set. Babies get their first teeth at around 6 months. Children begin to lose teeth at age 6. Adult teeth begin to come in at 6 or 7. They won't all be in until you turn 21!

Your DIGESTIVE TRACT

Your digestive tract is a long tube that extends from your mouth to your anus. Along the way there are special helper organs that send chemicals into the digestive tube. These chemicals help to digest or break down food into small particles. The small particles, called **nutrients,** are absorbed by small blood vessels in the walls of the digestive tube. The blood then carries the nutrients all over the body to each and every cell. The cells of the body use nutrients for energy and growth. Food that was not absorbed in the digestive tube keeps moving until it reaches the end and is expelled.

Start Here!

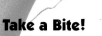
Go on a ride with your favorite food

Parotid gland
(saliva gland)

sublingual and Submandibular glands
(saliva gland)

S W A L L O W

1 Take a Bite!
Your teeth *chew and break food down into smaller pieces.* **Your tongue** *helps you talk, swallow and taste. It is made of muscles and is covered with thousands of taste buds.*

2 Get a Bath!
Your salivary glands *send* **saliva** *into your mouth to mix with food. Saliva is not just water. It is a special chemical fluid that begins digesting food and makes it easier to swallow.*

3 Enjoy the Ride!
Your throat *is about five inches long. Your air passage (trachea) and your throat both connect to your mouth. The epiglottis is like a door between your throat and the entrance to your air passage. It keeps food from going down the wrong tube. Once you swallow, the rest is automatic.*

4 Get Squeezed!
Your esophagus *is about ten inches long. Its muscular walls squeeze the food all the way down to your stomach.*

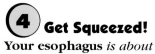
To the stomach

food moves from your mouth to your stomach in about 6 seconds

Your SPECIAL HELPER ORGANS

Your LIVER

Lots of Action!

The liver is a large helper organ connected to the digestive tube just past the stomach. The liver is like a factory. It makes **bile,** a chemical that helps digest fats. It makes chains of body proteins in food. The liver stores extra food energy until your body needs it. The liver cleans bad stuff out of the body, like drugs, alcohol and poisons.

6 Liver *makes bile and stores food energy*

7 Gallbladder *stores bile from liver*

Your STOMACH

Get All Mixed Up!

The stomach is a large curved part of the digestive tube. Its walls are very muscular and have lots of folds that stretch to hold food. Your food is mixed with **gastric juices** here. Gastric juices are acid chemicals made by the stomach. They digest food into small particles. Now your food is in liquid form. The stomach squirts it out into the small intestine a little at a time.

From the esophagus

5 Stomach *mixes food*

8 Pancreas *produces digestive juices*

9 Duodenum *connects the stomach with the intestines*

To the intestines

Your GALLBLADDER

Storage

The gallbladder is a small helper organ just under the liver. It stores bile made by the liver and sends it to the digestive tube when food passes by.

Your DUODENUM

Get Juiced!

The duodenum is the section of digestive tube that starts at the bottom of the stomach and ends at the top of your intestines. The liver, gallbladder and pancreas send their digestive juices into the duodenum to help break down the food into smaller particles and get it ready for the next step.

Your PANCREAS

Feel the Power!

The pancreas is a special helper organ that adds chemicals to the digestive tube. These chemicals help digest food and help your body use the energy in carbohydrates.

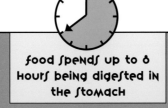

food spends up to 6 hours being digested in the stomach

Your SMALL INTESTINE Take a wild ride!

The small intestine is almost 25 feet long! Food is squeezed through while digestion continues. Absorption begins in the small intestine. The inside walls of your small intestine are covered with millions of tiny finger-like projections called **villi.** The villi help absorb nutrients. Absorbed nutrients then enter the blood stream and travel to all the cells of your body.

food spends up to 4 hours traveling through the small intestine.

6 Nutrients enter your cells. You have energy to work and grow!

5 The blood carries the nutrients to each cell in your body.

4 The usable nutrients are sent back into your blood vessels.

3 The liver processes the nutrients into particles your body can use.

2 These blood vessels carry the nutrients to your liver.

1 Nutrients are absorbed through the walls of your intestines into blood vessels inside.

Follow nutrients as they travel through the body!

Villi
Blood vessel
Nutrients

11 Large Intestine

ABSORB WATER

DIGEST

AND

ABSORB NUTRIENTS

Small Intestine
10

IF YOU STRETCH OUT ALL THE VILLI IN THE SMALL INTESTINE AND FLATTEN THEM, THEY WOULD COVER A TENNIS COURT!

YOUR LARGE INTESTINE STARTS HERE.

STORE WASTE

food spends up to 12 hours in the Large intestine while water is absorbed.

The **appendix** *is attached to the large intestine. It has no function in our bodies today. Some people think it was once an extra stomach!*

The **rectum** *stores unused parts of food you eat and bacteria that live in your intestines. They leave the body as feces, the solid waste of the digestive process.*

12

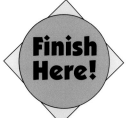

Finish Here!

Your LARGE INTESTINE
Hang out for a while...

The large intestine is about five feet long. It has lots of folds and pouches to hold food wastes. The unused part of your food is stored while the water in it is absorbed back into your body.

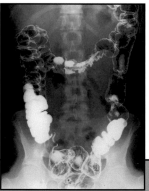

Here is an x-ray of the large intestine. Can you see the appendix?

activities

WHAT ARE CALORIES?

A calorie is the measure of how much energy is in food. Some foods have lots of calories in them, some have a little. If there aren't enough calories in the food you eat, your body will not have the energy it needs to run well. If there are too many calories, the extra will be stored as fat.

WHERE DOES GAS COME FROM?

You are not alone! There are millions of friendly bacteria living in your intestines. They eat tiny amounts of the parts of food you can't absorb. When bacteria digest this fiber, they give off gas, which collects in your intestines until it is...released.

WHY DO I THROW UP?

When something bad gets in your stomach, or when you are feeling ill, your stomach will get rid of whatever is in it. To do this, the stomach closes off its lower exit, opens the upper entrance, and with a big squeeze of its muscular walls, forces everything backward up your esophagus.

WHAT IS A BURP?

Sometimes air is trapped in your stomach from swallowing or from gas that is made when food is broken down by gastric juices. This air or gas collects at the top of your stomach until suddenly it is released, making a sound as it goes up your throat and out your mouth!

HIGH FIVE FOR FOOD!

Name your FINGERS!

One for every food group

Mark an **X** in a square for each serving you eat. Try to fill up to your fingertips every day!

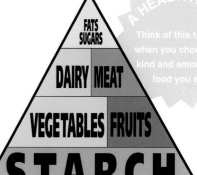

DAIRY
STARCH
FRUIT
VEGGIES
MEAT

Limit your servings of fats and sugars. They have calories, but not as many nutrients as the five major food groups.

The Right Way to Brush

Brush for at least three minutes twice a day.

Time yourself!

Start at the gums with your brush tilted. Brush toward tips of the teeth

Brush all surfaces and Floss every day.

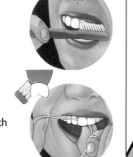

A HEALTHY DIET
Think of this triangle when you choose the kind and amounts of food you eat.

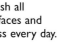

FATS SUGARS

DAIRY MEAT

VEGETABLES FRUITS

STARCH

Eating the right foods gives you a healthy balance of all these important nutrients.

PROTEINS	CARBOHYDRATES	FATS	FIBER	VITAMINS & MINERALS	WATER
Proteins are the body's building blocks. Nearly everything in the body has protein in it. Protein is found in meat, eggs, poultry, fish, nuts and beans.	Carbohydrates are your body's main source of energy. They are found in starchy vegetables and fruits, potatoes, rice, pasta, breads, and sugars.	Fats are used by the body to make parts of each cell. Fat is also a very powerful source of energy. Fat is found in meats, milk, cheese, eggs, butter, vegetable oils and nuts.	Fiber keeps your digestion running smoothly. Some is digested and helps balance the nutrients in your blood. The rest is eliminated at the end of digestion. Fiber is found in fresh fruits and vegetables.	Vitamins and minerals act as messengers and helpers inside your cells. They help change food into energy and keep your body healthy. They are found in most foods in very small amounts.	Your body's cells are made of over half water! Water is an important part of your blood, saliva, and other body fluids. Your body needs water to work well, so drink 6 to 8 glasses a day.

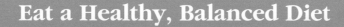

Eat a Healthy, Balanced Diet

Your EYES

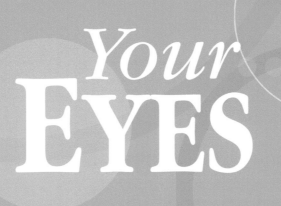

FUN FACTS

- Your retina is only as thick as a piece of paper.
- The eye can see 7 to 10 million different colors.
- Your eyeball is an extension of your brain!
- Your eye turns the light you see into electricity. The electricity is the signal sent to your brain.
- Birds see many more colors than humans can.
- Bees can see things that are invisible to us, because they can see ultraviolet light and polarized light, two kinds of light we can't see.
- Snakes can see heat. They can see infrared light, which we feel as heat.
- Hawks can see 6 times further than humans can.
- Frogs can see more colors than dogs can.
- You average 6 blinks a minute or over 3 million blinks a year!

Your EYES

You collect huge amounts of information about the world with your eyes. Your eyes send it to your brain to be decoded and processed. Your brain helps make sense of the world your eyes see.

Tears from your **lacrimal gland** *clean dust and germs out of your eye. They wash over your eyes and drain out through the* **pores,** *then down little canals to the* **lacrimal sac.** *They travel through the* **nasolacrimal duct** *and out through your nose. That's why your nose runs when you cry!*

Eye PROTECTION

Eyebrows, eyelashes, eyelids and tears all protect your eyes. Your eyebrows catch dirt and sweat, and your eyelashes trap dust. They both help keep out the sun. Your eyelids protect and cover your eyeballs.

Eye MUSCLES

Six eye muscles on the outside of each eyeball work together to move your eye. They help keep your eye round and inside your head!

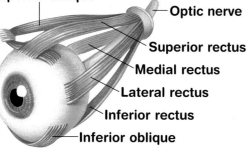

Superior oblique

Optic nerve

Superior rectus

Medial rectus

Lateral rectus

Inferior rectus

Inferior oblique

TOO bright or TOO dark?

Your eye regulates how much light you see. Muscles in your **iris** relax or contract automatically, changing the size of the **pupil**, the dark center in your eye.

Iris

In bright light, your pupil is tiny. The muscle in your iris contracts.

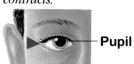

When light is dim, your pupil gets larger to let more light in.

Pupil

Inside your
EYES

Your eye is filled with very special fluids called humors.

The back of each eye is filled with a jelly-like humor called **vitreous humor.** This fluid helps keep your eyeball round and keeps the lens and retina in place.

In front of the lens is a watery fluid called **aqueous humor.** It carries nutrients to the cornea.

Your fovea is the point of sharpest focus for light on your retina. There are lots of cones here.

Your optic disc is where all the nerves from the retina join together in your optic nerve.

This is your "blind spot." There are no rods or cones here.

*The **optic nerve** is made of nerve fibers from the **retina** that joined together at the back of the eye. The optic nerve takes information directly to the brain.*

Anatomy of the Eye

The **lens** is a round, flat and perfectly clear structure that bends the light as it shines through it. It helps you focus. The lens has many layers just like an onion. Your lens gets bigger throughout your life!

The **sclera** is the "white of the eye." This tough, protective layer keeps the eyeball round.

The **cornea** is the perfectly clear, front part of the eye. It allows light to pass into the eye. Its curved surface bends light rays entering your eye.

The **iris** is the colored part of your eye. Its dark center is actually an opening, called the **pupil.**

The **ciliary body** is a muscular ring that lies just behind the iris. It has tiny fibers that attach to the lens. The ciliary muscles pull on the fibers attached to the lens, changing the lens shape to help focus light.

The **choroid** has lots of blood vessels. It stores nutrients and Vitamin A for the retina. Its deep brown pigment absorbs and keeps light from bouncing all over the inside of your eyeball.

Your
RETINA

The retina is actually inside out! Light passes all the way through it before reaching the light-sensing cells at the back of it!

The signal made there passes from cell to cell and then out to your optic nerve and brain.

To optic nerve

Signal out

Light in

Rod

Cone

Photograph of the Retina

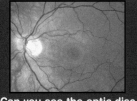

Can you see the optic disc in this photograph?
Where is the fovea, the point of sharpest vision?

Your
RODS AND CONES

Your retina has special cells that sense the light entering your eye—

Rods are tall, skinny cells. They are most sensitive to dim light and they sense only shades of gray. They are our night vision receptors. You have 125 million rods in each eye!

Cones are color vision receptors. There are blue, red, and green cones. The three kinds of cone cells each detect a different color of light. You see colors like pink and purple when combinations of cones are excited. You have 1 million cones in each eye!

Seeing the light

Light Waves!

The light waves we see are a small part of the **ELECTROMAGNETIC RADIATION SPECTRUM** (shown below). This spectrum not only includes light waves that we use to see, but also gamma rays, X-Rays, ultraviolet waves, infrared waves, microwaves and radio waves.

VISIBLE LIGHT, the waves we can see, are split into colors. Objects have color because they absorb some of this visible light spectrum and reflect the rest. We see the color that objects reflect.

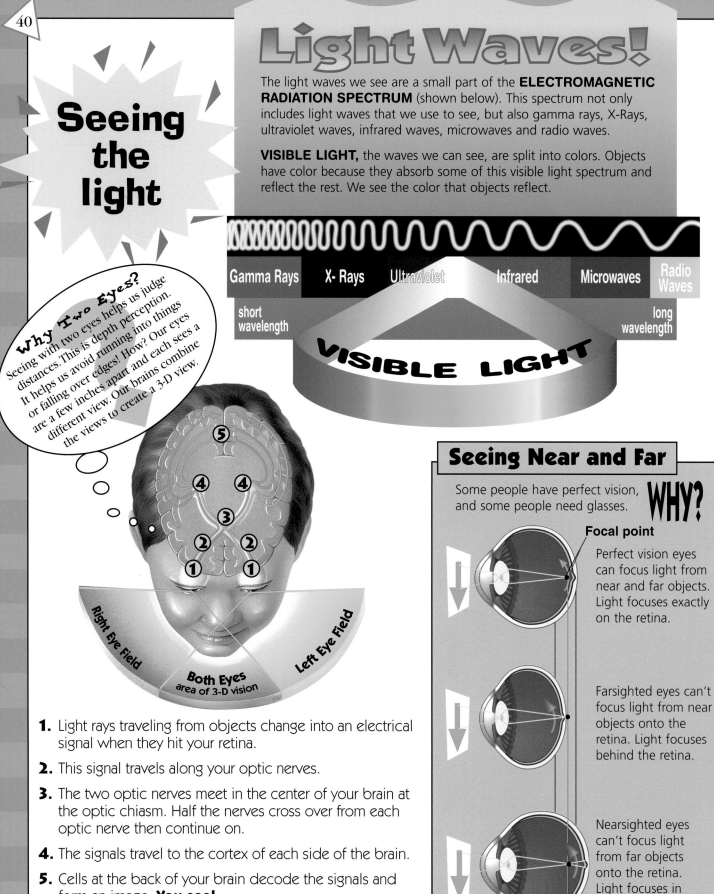

| Gamma Rays | X- Rays | Ultraviolet | Infrared | Microwaves | Radio Waves |

short wavelength

long wavelength

VISIBLE LIGHT

Why Two Eyes?

Seeing with two eyes helps us judge distances. This is depth perception. It helps us avoid running into things or falling over edges! How? Our eyes are a few inches apart and each sees a different view. Our brains combine the views to create a 3-D view.

Right Eye Field

Left Eye Field

Both Eyes
area of 3-D vision

1. Light rays traveling from objects change into an electrical signal when they hit your retina.

2. This signal travels along your optic nerves.

3. The two optic nerves meet in the center of your brain at the optic chiasm. Half the nerves cross over from each optic nerve then continue on.

4. The signals travel to the cortex of each side of the brain.

5. Cells at the back of your brain decode the signals and form an image. **You see!**

Seeing Near and Far

Some people have perfect vision, and some people need glasses. **WHY?**

Focal point

Perfect vision eyes can focus light from near and far objects. Light focuses exactly on the retina.

Farsighted eyes can't focus light from near objects onto the retina. Light focuses behind the retina.

Nearsighted eyes can't focus light from far objects onto the retina. Light focuses in front of the retina.

Glasses are man-made lenses. They bend the light, which moves the focal point onto the retina. This helps eyes correctly focus light on the retina.

activities

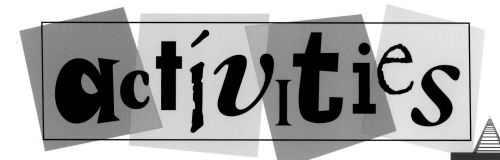

Which red box is bigger?

Careful! You can be fooled by pictures like this one. Visual tricks can create the appearance of depth. Since the blue lines look like they go off into the distance, the top red box looks farther away. And it goes all the way across the "track." These visual clues make the top box seem bigger.

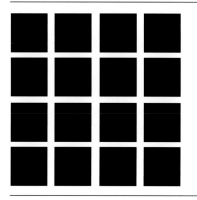

See spots before your eyes!

Do you see the gray spots between the squares? Some of your retina cells get over-excited by the criss-crossing white lines. Then they signal your brain that there's NO light coming in at that spot! Your eyes and brain are confused by the white and black areas so close together.

Color ghosts!

Stare at the center of the red circle for 30 seconds. Then quickly stare at a blank white surface. What do you see? The green ghost-like circle you see on the blank page is a color "after-image." This happens when the red cone cells in your eye get "tired," or over-stimulated, as you stare at the red circle. When you look away, only the green and blue cones are working well enough to make an image of the circle, which appears to be on the blank page, but it is actually on your retina.

Find your blind spot!

Stand at arm's length from this page. Close your left eye.

Look at the red O.

Move your head forward until the blue X disappears.

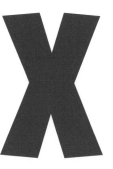

Everyone has a blind spot! There are no rods or cones in your optic disc, where your optic nerve fibers leave the back of your eye. You don't usually notice this blank area because your brain fills it in with information from your other eye.

Your EARS

FUN FACTS

➤ Sound travels 4 times faster in water than in air!

➤ The lowest note you can hear, a low rumble, vibrates at 20 times a second. The highest note, a high hiss, vibrates at 20,000 times a second!

➤ For you to be able to hear a sound, your eardrum has to move only 40 billionths of an inch!

➤ Light travels 100,000 times faster than sound! That's why we see lightning before we hear thunder!

➤ The smallest bones in the body are in your ear.

➤ Humans can hear sounds from very faint whispers to sounds one million times as loud!

➤ At room temperature, sound waves travel over 1,000 feet per second!

Your EARS
Hearing and Balance

*The **outer ear** or **pinna** is just a small part of your whole ear, the part you can see!*

Your BALANCE

Your sense of balance is a warning system. It lets you know if you are unstable or about to stumble.

*Balance begins in the **semicircular canals** and **vestibule** of the inner ear.*

Your inner ear is filled with fluids and stones! When they move, nerves send signals about the position of your head to the brain.

*Your **semicircular canals** track movement, like twirling around or rolling upside down. Each canal lies in a different direction, one for front–back, up–down, or left–right, the 3 dimensions of space.*

Cupola

*At the base of the canals are fluid-filled little rooms, or **ampullae.***

*When you move, the fluid moves and bends the **cupola**. Nerves connected to it send signals to the brain.*

Cupola

*The **vestibule** tracks gravity when you are still but your surroundings are moving, like riding in a car.*

Otoliths, *or "ear stones," lie at the bottom of sacs in the vestibule.*

Hair Cells

Nerve

Ampulla

Vestibule

Cochlea

Hair Cells

Nerve

When your head moves, little hairs in the sacs are bent by the weight of the stones. Nerves connected to the hairs signal your brain about head position.

Animals like DOGS, CATS and DEER can swivel their ears freely! Moveable ears catch more sound and help pinpoint the location of the sound.

Frogs can hear just the range of sounds that their fellow frogs make! A frog's eardrum is on the outside of its head. The eardrum is attached to only one bone, not three, as in humans.

Inside your
EARS

The **middle ear** starts behind the eardrum. It is home to the ear bones: the hammer, anvil and stirrup, or **malleus, incus and stapes.** The malleus connects to the eardrum, then to the incus and the stapes. The base of the stapes rests on the oval window.

The **inner ear** lies deep in your skull bone. It is called the **labyrinth,** meaning maze. It's made of three curved channels called the **semicircular canals**, the **vestibule,** and a snail-like coil called the **cochlea.** These curving spaces inside your skull are filled with fluid.

Here's a view of the eardrum looking down the ear canal, as a doctor sees it! Can you see the shadow where the malleus attaches to the eardrum?

Two nerves collect the signals from your inner ear and send them to the brain.

The **vestibular nerve** *sends information about balance. The* **cochlear nerve** *sends information about sound.*

Inner Ear

Middle Ear

Semi-circular canals

Bone

Vestibular nerve

Cochlear nerve

Outer Ear

Malleus

Incus

Vestibule

Your cochlea is the size of a pea. It senses sound through fluid movement.

Cochlea

The **ear canal** *reaches through the skull bone to the middle ear. The skin lining the ear canal makes ear wax, or* **cebum.**

Eardrum

Stapes

Oval window

The **round window** *at the end of the cochlea is the safety pressure valve for the inner ear.*

Cartilage *under the skin gives the outer ear its funny shape. The shape helps direct sound down your ear canal to the eardrum.*

The **eardrum** *is 1/3" wide, and 1/50" thick, as thin as paper! It is covered with a thin layer of skin. The eardrum is attached to the malleus. When the eardrum moves, the malleus moves, transmitting sound vibrations to the inner ear.*

The 1-1/2" long **auditory tube** *connects the middle ear to your throat. It acts as a pressure equalizer and safety valve for the middle ear.*

WHY DO YOUR EARS POP?

To hear, your eardrum has to vibrate. Air pressure on either side must be equal or the eardrum won't vibrate. When outside pressure changes, pressure inside the middle ear must equalize, or match outside pressure. Your auditory tube lets air in and out of the middle ear. The tube is usually narrow. When you swallow or yawn the tube opens and air rushes in. The "pop" is the feeling of pressure equalizing, and your eardrum moving again!

HOW LOUD IS LOUD?

Loudness or intensity of sound is measured in **decibels.**

0 decibels

10 decibels — A pin drop

20 decibels — A whisper

50 decibels — Normal conversation

70 decibels — Traffic or restaurant noise - loud, but not harmful.

90-100 decibels — Lawn mower, loud music, kids screaming on a playground! Over time can cause hearing damage.

120 decibels — Speakers at a rock concert. This can cause permanent hearing loss.

Crickets have simple ears on their legs! They can hear only a small range of sounds, mostly those of other crickets.

BATS use their ears to steer! In the dark, they make sounds that bounce off of objects nearby. The returning echoes tell the size and position of the object. Bats can find objects as thin as a hair this way!

Your HEADING

Your HEARING

Hearing sound is all about movement -movement of air, membranes, bones, fluids and hairs! The energy of sound waves is turned into electrical signals to the brain!

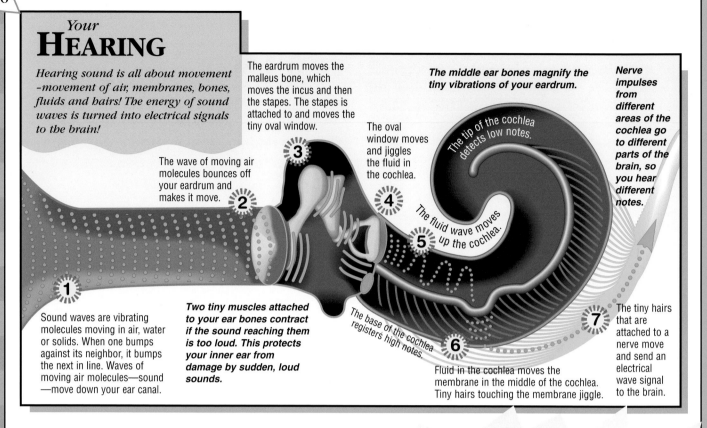

The eardrum moves the malleus bone, which moves the incus and then the stapes. The stapes is attached to and moves the tiny oval window.

The middle ear bones magnify the tiny vibrations of your eardrum.

Nerve impulses from different areas of the cochlea go to different parts of the brain, so you hear different notes.

The wave of moving air molecules bounces off your eardrum and makes it move.

The oval window moves and jiggles the fluid in the cochlea.

The tip of the cochlea detects low notes.

The fluid wave moves up the cochlea.

3

2

4

5

The base of the cochlea registers high notes.

1

Sound waves are vibrating molecules moving in air, water or solids. When one bumps against its neighbor, it bumps the next in line. Waves of moving air molecules—sound —move down your ear canal.

Two tiny muscles attached to your ear bones contract if the sound reaching them is too loud. This protects your inner ear from damage by sudden, loud sounds.

6

7

The tiny hairs that are attached to a nerve move and send an electrical wave signal to the brain.

Fluid in the cochlea moves the membrane in the middle of the cochlea. Tiny hairs touching the membrane jiggle.

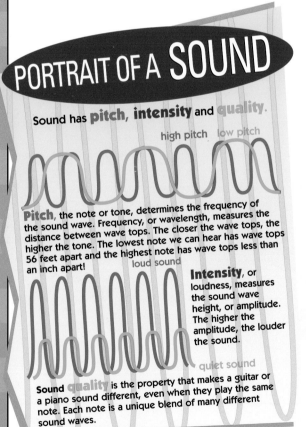

PORTRAIT OF A SOUND

Sound has **pitch**, **intensity** and **quality**.

high pitch   low pitch

Pitch, the note or tone, determines the frequency of the sound wave. Frequency, or wavelength, measures the distance between wave tops. The closer the wave tops, the higher the tone. The lowest note we can hear has wave tops 56 feet apart and the highest note has wave tops less than an inch apart!

loud sound

Intensity, or loudness, measures the sound wave height, or amplitude. The higher the amplitude, the louder the sound.

quiet sound

Sound quality is the property that makes a guitar or a piano sound different, even when they play the same note. Each note is a unique blend of many different sound waves.

Listen Up!
EAR PROBLEMS

- Loud noises can make you go deaf! Repeated loud sounds, such as loud rock music or heavy machinery, can damage the hair cells in your cochlea. Some musicians lose some hearing after years of listening to their own loud music.

- Don't blow your nose too hard! Blowing too hard can force mucus and germs up your auditory tube and cause a middle ear infection.

- A bad cold can cause temporary hearing loss. Your auditory tube swells shut and can't open to equalize pressure behind the eardrum. The eardrum can't move, so you can't hear. As you recover, your hearing improves.

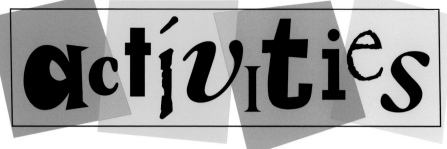

activities

Locating Sound

1. Blindfold a friend (this is the fun part).
2. Have your friend cover one ear.
3. Tap two pencils together.
4. Ask your friend to point to where the sound is coming from.
5. How often is your friend correct with one ear uncovered? With both ears uncovered?

What happens?
We locate sound better using two ears because we detect a tiny difference in arrival time of the sound at each ear.

Make an EARDRUM you can see!

1. Stretch a plastic bag tightly over the top of a can and fasten it on with a rubber band.
2. Sprinkle sugar on the stretched plastic.
3. Bang a metal handle on the edge of the can.

What happens?
When the sound waves travel from the metal can to the stretched plastic, they move the plastic, and the sugar bounces!

MAKE A WALKIE TALKIE!

1. You'll need two tin cans and a few feet of string. Punch a hole in the ends of the cans, pull the string through and knot it inside each can.

2. Give one can to a friend. Stretch the string out tight and take turns talking quietly and listening through the cans.

What's happening?
The string is vibrated by the sound of your voice, and the sound wave moves down the string to your friend's can.

Why am I so loud?
Sounds made in your head, such as speaking or chewing, seem much louder to you than to those around you. **Why?** Your own voice vibrates solid objects (like your skull bones) inside your head and sound travels to your ears.

What are "the spins"?
When you spin around really fast, the fluid in your semicircular canals spins too. When you stop, the fluid keeps spinning. Your brain thinks you are still spinning, but your eyes tell your brain you've stopped. When your ears catch up with your eyes you stop feeling dizzy.

Why can we hear under water?
Moving water molecules transfer sound to our ears just as air molecules do.

Why do you have EAR WAX?
It protects your ear by trapping dust and bugs before they get to the delicate eardrum.

Can you WIGGLE your ears?
Some people can! There are tiny muscles behind the ear flap, but most people can't control them very well.

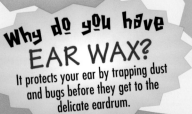

Your TASTE *and* SMELL

FUN FACTS

➤ Hot foods such as chili peppers excite pain receptors and taste receptors in your mouth.

➤ Flies taste with their feet! They have taste receptors on their feet as well as their mouths.

➤ Sharks can smell 1 part blood to 1 million parts water! Human olfactory bulbs are quite small, but a shark's are the biggest part of it's brain.

➤ A dog's sense of smell is up to 100 million times better than a human's! Dogs have 15 square inches of olfactory epithelium, compared to our 1 1/2 inches!!!

➤ Albino animals have no sense of smell. Normally the pigments that color skin are also in olfactory epithelium, and help the sense of smell. An albino animal has no pigment so the sense of smell is absent.

➤ A taste bud lasts about 10 days before it is replaced.

➤ After age 75, the number of taste buds starts to decrease.

Your TASTE and SMELL

Taste and Smell are two special parts of your nervous system called the "*chemical senses*". They detect particles found in fluids, either in saliva or in the moist lining of your nose. Taste and smell work together. When your nose is plugged, food seems to lose its taste. That's because 80% of the flavor of food comes from your sense of smell.

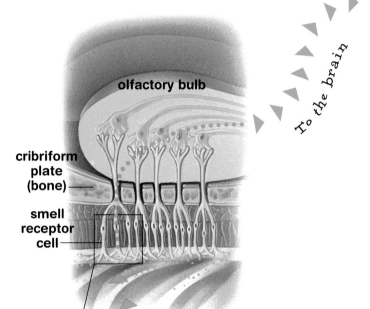

olfactory bulb

cribriform plate (bone)

smell receptor cell

To the brain

3 The smell receptor cells send signals up their fibers. The signals pass through tiny holes in the bony **cribriform plate**.

2 ...then the particles attach to hairs on **smell receptor cells** lying in the mucus.

1 Tiny particles in the air you breathe dissolve in the **mucus** lining in your nose...

smell receptor cell

mucus

Even though olfactory **smell receptor cells** are in your nose, they are actually part of your brain! These nerve cells are in direct contact with the outside world. Unlike any other nervous tissue in your body, they can regrow. Each one lasts about a month before it is replaced by a fresh cell.

What smells are special to you? Baking cookies? Newly cut grass? Your grandma's house? Smells can bring back memories and feelings. Your olfactory nerves are connected to a part of your brain that also influences emotion and memory!

How you smell things

Inside your
NOSE *and* MOUTH

6 *Smell centers in your brain process the signal.*

5 *...and travels through your brain along the* **olfactory tract.**

4 *The signal reaches the* **olfactory bulb**...

▶ ▶ ▶ ▶ ▶ ▶ ▶

From the
smell receptors

The **olfactory epithelium**, *or "smelling skin", is only about 1-1/2 square inches, but it has over 15 million receptor cells!*

Taste signals pass through several specialized areas on the way to the cortex. This outer part of your brain processes the signal.

4

3

Three nerves carry taste signals from the taste buds on your tongue to your brain.

◀ ◀ ◀ ◀
◀
◀
◀
◀
◀
◀

Anatomy of a
SNIFF

Air takes a crooked path through your nose. small bones called **conchae** narrow and twist your nasal passage. Usually only 2% of your breath reaches your **olfactory epithelium**. But take a **BIG** sniff! More air travels higher—more scent particles reach the smell sensors at the top of your nasal passage.

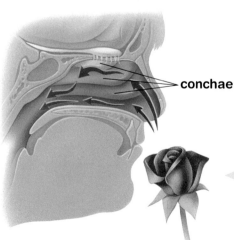

conchae

Your tongue is made of several muscles joined together. Can you think of at least 4 different uses for your tongue?

▲
▲
▲
▲

Your
TONGUE

Bumps and buds!

Your tongue is covered with bumps called **papillae**.

Look for these 4 kinds of papillae on your tongue! Three have taste buds and one is rough for scraping and licking.

Vallate papillae
are 7-12 large bumps at the back of your tongue. 250 taste buds are hidden in each valley.

Filliform papillae
are tiny, file-shaped bumps that scrape and clean. Though these are the most numerous papillae, they have no taste buds.

Fungiform papillae
are mushroom-shaped bumps on the top and sides of your tongue that contain taste buds.

Foliate papillae
are leaf-shaped bumps on each side of your tongue near the back that contain taste buds.

1,000 times life-size

2 *Each taste bud has several* **taste receptor cells**. *Tiny hairs reach out through a hole at the top of the taste bud. The dissolved food particles attach to these hairs. This sends a a signal up the receptor cell nerve fiber.*

To the brain

1 *Tiny particles from food dissolve into your* **saliva**. *Saliva coats the* **taste buds** *on your tongue's papillae. You have over 10,000 taste buds on the papillae of your tongue and scattered around the inside of your mouth.*

How you taste things

Types of Tongues

A **snake's** tongue acts like a nose! It flicks out to catch smells as they go by on the breeze.

A **chameleon's** tongue has a sticky tip to grab and hold insects.

An **anteater's** tongue is almost a yard! This insect eater catches bugs by snaking its tongue down insects nests.

A **dog** uses its tongue to cool off! When a dog pants, moisture evaporates off its tongue. This process cools down its whole body.

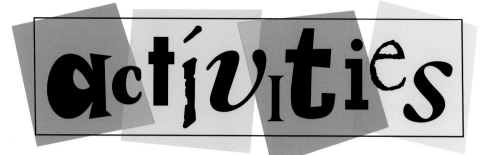

activities

THE NOSE KNOWS

1. Blindfold a friend.
2. Have her taste small cubes of first an apple and then a raw potato.
3. Ask her to identify what she tastes. *How does she do?*
4. Ask her to hold her nose and repeat the test. *How does she do with her nose plugged? Why?*

Make a Tongue Map!

With a friend, map out the taste regions on your tongue.

1. Make 4 solutions: add 1 teaspoon flavoring each to a 1/2 cup of water: sugar (sweet), salt (salty), lemon juice (bitter), vinegar (sour).
2. Touch a cotton swab first to a solution and then to different areas on your friend's tongue.
3. Mark the areas that respond to each flavor on a drawing of a tongue. Then trade places. *Are your maps the same?*

nose plugged? Why?

Tricky Taste!

1. Blindfold a friend.
2. Hold an onion under his nose while he tastes a piece of apple. *What does he think he is eating? Why?*

Taste Territory

- You sense 4 basic tastes. Every flavor, like 'pickle', is a combination of these 4 tastes.

- Each taste bud can sense all of these tastes, but is most sensitive to one.

- Your bitter receptors are most sensitive, then sour, then sweet and salt.

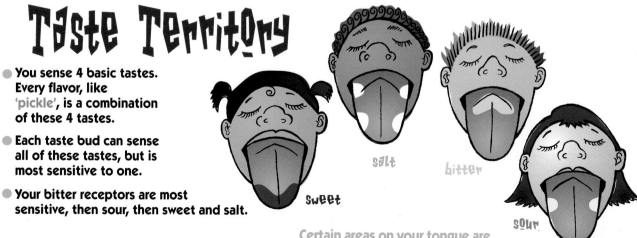

sweet salt bitter sour

Certain areas on your tongue are most sensitive to one of the 4 basic tastes.

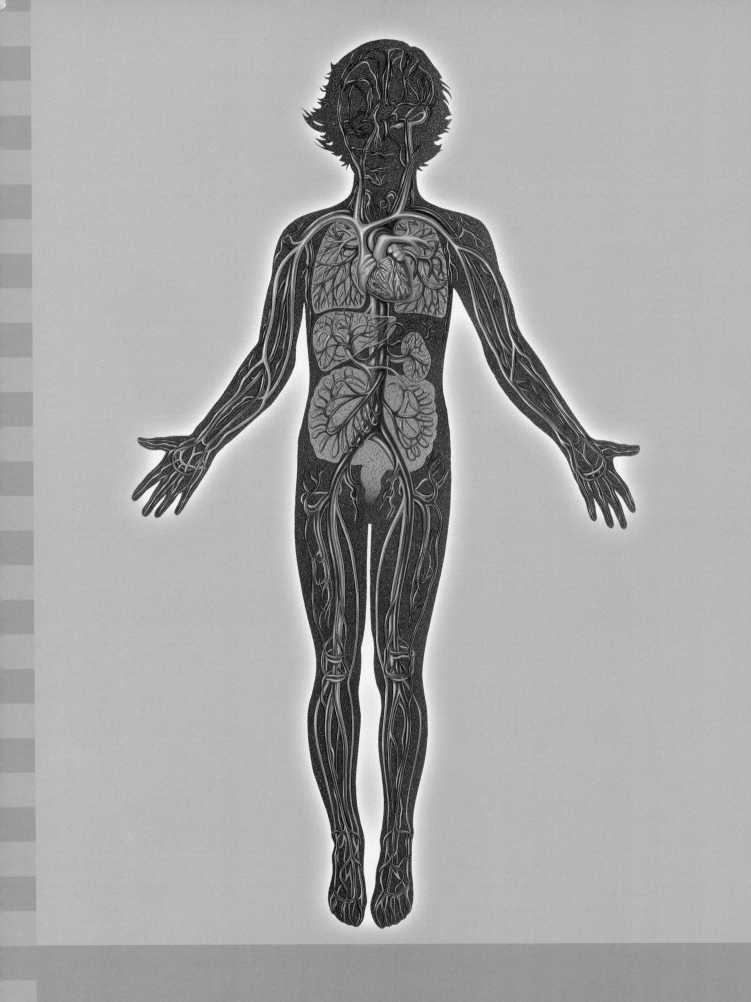

GLOSSARY

AORTA
The large arterial blood vessel that carries blood from the left ventricle out to the body.

ARTERY
A blood vessel that carries blood away from the heart.

ATRIUM
One of two upper chambers in the heart.

BICEPS
Muscle found in the upper part of the arm.

BORBORYGMUS
The rumbling noise made by gas and fluids moving in the intestines.

BRONCHIOLE
Small airway passages that branch off of the main airway passage, bronchus, in the lung.

BRONCHUS
Large airway passages that brings air into the lungs.

CAPILLARY
Very small blood vessels that connect arteries to veins.

CARBON DIOXIDE
A gas produced by our cells as a waste product that is exhaled into the air.

CEREBELLUM
The part of the brain that controls movement.

CEREBRUM
The largest part of the brain, thinking part, divided into a left and right hemisphere.

COCCYX
The bone at the end of your spine, also called the tail bone.

CORNEA
The clear part of the eye where light enters so you can see.

DIAPHRAGM
The muscular sheet that lies under the lung cavity, dividing your chest and abdomen area. It helps you breathe.

DIGESTION
A process that breaks down food into tiny particles so it can be absorbed into the blood stream.

EPIGLOTTIS
A structure behind the tongue that prevents food from entering the larynx.

ESOPHAGUS
Another name for the "throat," a muscular tube that connects the mouth to the stomach.

FOCAL POINT
The spot where light entering the eye focuses.

INTESTINE
The tubular part of the digestive system between your stomach and the anus that absorbs nutrients and water.

IRIS
The colored part of your eye just behind your cornea.

JOINT
The place where two or more bones meet. Some joints are movable (shoulder) and others are not (between skull bones).

LACRIMAL GLAND
A gland above the eye that produces tears.

LARYNX
The structure located on top of the windpipe, also called the voice box.

MANDIBLE
Jaw bone.

MARROW
The soft, spongy material that fills the center of long bones.

NERVE CELL
A long cell that is the functional unit of the nervous system.

NUTRIENT
The part of food that the body uses for energy.

OXYGEN
A gas in the air we breathe in and our bodies use to release energy.

PATELLA
The bone located in front of and between our upper and lower leg, also called the knee cap.

SALIVA
Fluid released by salivary glands of the mouth that digests food.

TENDON
A tough tissue that connects muscle to bone.

TISSUE
A group of cells that work together for a particular function.

VEIN
A blood vessel that carries blood towards the heart.

VERTEBRA
One of the bones of the spine.

Blueprints for Health
REFERENCES

Allison, Linda. Blood and Guts. Covelo, CO: Yolla Bolly, 1976.

Anderson, Karen C., and Stephen Cumbaa. The Bones and Skeleton Game Book. New York: Workman, 1993.

Ardley, Neil. The Science Book of the Senses. San Diego: Harcourt Brace, 1992.

Bailey, Frederick. Bailey's Textbook of Histology. Baltimore: Williams & Wilkins, 1978.

Campbell, Neil A. Biology, 3rd ed. Redwood City, CA: Benjamin-Cummings, 1993.

Caselli, Giovanni. The Human Body and How It Works. London: Dorling Kindersley, 1992.

Cassin, Sue, and David Smith. Fascinating Facts About Your Body. New York: Warner, 1989.

Clayman, Charles B., The Human Body. New York: Dorling Kindersley, 1995.

Cumbaa, Stephen. The Bones Book and Skeleton. New York: Workman, 1991.

Day, Trevor. The Random House Book of 1001 Questions and Answers About the Human Body. New York: Random House, 1994.

Ganeri, Anita. The Usborne Book of Body Facts. London: Usborne Publishing Limited, 1992.

Goodman, Susan. Amazing Biofacts. New York: P. Bedrick Books, 1993.

Grant, J.C. Boileau. Grant's Atlas of Anatomy. Baltimore: Williams and Wilkins, 1983.

Hindley, Judy. How Your Body Works. London: Usborne Publishing Limited, 1988.

Kaufman, Joe. The Human Body. Racine, Wisc.: Western Publishing, 1987.

Kessel, Richard G. Tissues and Organs. New York: W. H. Freeman, 1979.

Marieb, Elaine N. Human Anatomy and Physiology, 2nd ed. Redwood City, CA: Benjamin-Cummings, 1992.

National Geographic Society. The Incredible Machine. Washington, D.C.: National Geographic Society, 1986.

National Geographic Society. Your Wonderful Body. Washington, D.C.: National Geographic Society, 1982.

Netter, Frank H. Atlas of Human Anatomy. West Caldwell, NJ: CIBA-GEIGY, 1989.

Nourse, Alan E., and the editors of Life. The Body. New York: Time Inc., 1664

Parker, Steve. The Body Atlas. London: Dorling Kindersley, 1993.

Parker, Steve. How the Body Works. New York: RD Association, 1994.

Parker, Steve. The Random House Book of How Nature Works. New York: Random House, 1993.

Platzer, Werner, M.D. Pernkopf Anatomy: Atlas of Topographic and Applied Human Anatomy, 3rd ed., 2 vols., Trans. Harry Monsen. Baltimore: Urban & Schwarzenberg, 1989.

Royston, Angela. The Human Body and How It Works. New York: Random House, 1991.

Seddon, Tony. Investigating Me. New York: Derrydale Books., 1991.

Stein, Sara B. The Body Book. New York: Workman, 1992.

Stidworthy, John. Animal Biology. New York: Prentice Hall, 1992.

Suzuki, David T. Looking at the Body. New York: Wiley, 1991.

Whitfield, Philip, and Mike Stoddart. The Human Body. Tarrytown, NY: Torstar, 1984.

Williams, Peter L., Roger Warwick, M.D., Mary Dyson, and Lawrence Bannister. Gray's Anatomy, 37th ed. Edinburgh: Churchill Livingstone, 1989.